How to Write Your Nursing Dissertation

How to Write Your Nursing Dissertation

Edited by

Alan Glasper

Professor of Nursing and Programme Lead
Faculty of Health Sciences
University of Southampton, UK

Colin Rees

Lecturer
School of Nursing and Midwifery Studies
Cardiff University, UK

WILEY-BLACKWELL

A John Wiley & Sons, Ltd., Publication

Library of Congress Cataloging-in-Publication Data

Glasper, Edward Alan.
  How to write your nursing dissertation / Alan Glasper, Colin Rees.
      p. ; cm.
  Includes bibliographical references and index.
  ISBN 978-1-118-41071-4 (pbk. : alk. paper)
  I. Rees, Colin.   II. Title.
  [DNLM: 1. Dissertations, Academic as Topic.   2. Writing.   3. Evidence-Based Nursing.   WZ 345]
  808.06′661–dc23

                                                  2012025030

A catalogue record for this book is available from the British Library.

Wiley also publishes its books in a variety of electronic formats. Some content that appears in print may not be available in electronic books.

Cover design by Meaden Creative

Set in 9.5/12pt Minion by SPi Publishers Services, Pondicherry, India
Printed in Singapore by Ho Printing Singapore Pte Ltd

2   2013

Contents

List of Contributors, xiii

Foreword by Professor Carl May, xvi

Preface, xviii

About the companion website, xix

Acknowledgements, xx

The scenarios, xxi

Section 1 Starting your dissertation journey, 1

1 Starting your dissertation journey, 3
  Sheila Reading

  What are dissertations?, 3
  What are the features of a degree education?, 6
  Features of a dissertation, 8
  Planning your dissertation – essential considerations, 9
  Completing your dissertation and gaining a good classification, 11
  References, 12
  Further reading, 13

2 Introduction to writing your evidence-based practice dissertation, 14
  Alan Glasper and Colin Rees

  Sample guidelines for students undertaking an undergraduate
    healthcare dissertation, 14
  Typical learning outcomes for an undergraduate evidence-based
    practice dissertation, 15
  The dissertation, 16
  Guidelines for students undertaking an undergraduate evidence-based
    practice dissertation, 17

Typical postgraduate evidence-based practice dissertation module learning outcomes, **18**
Conclusion, **22**

3 Clinical effectiveness and evidence-based practice: background and history, **23**
Alan Glasper and Colin Rees

Introduction, **23**
Historical aspects of evidence-based practice, **24**
The contribution of the nursing profession to evidence-based practice, **25**
How is evidence sourced?, **26**
Conclusion, **27**
References, **27**

4 What is evidence-based practice and clinical effectiveness?, **29**
Andrée le May

Clinical effectiveness, **29**
Evidence-based practice, **33**
Making care more effective, **34**
References, **38**

5 The challenges of delivering practice based on best evidence (in primary, secondary and tertiary settings), **40**
Andrée le May

An evidence base for practice, **40**
Barriers to the use of research evidence in practice, **42**
Encouraging the use of research evidence in practice, **45**
Conclusion, **49**
References, **49**

Section 2 Sourcing and accessing evidence for your dissertation, 53

6 Sourcing the best evidence, **55**
Paul Boagy, Pat Maier and Alan Glasper

Exploring and refining your question, **55**
Searching for research articles, **59**
Devising your search strategy, **62**
Accessing journal literature, **65**
The Cochrane Library, **66**
Websites and other resources, **69**

Support from your library service, **70**
RCN information literacy competencies, **72**
Conclusion, **75**
References, **76**

7 What is grey literature and where can it be found?, **77**
   Alan Glasper and Colin Rees

   What is 'grey literature'?, **77**
   Where can I find grey literature?, **78**
   Important websites, **79**
   What about Google scholar?, **79**
   References, **79**

8 Harvard or Vancouver – getting it right all the time, **80**
   Alan Glasper and Colin Rees

   Vancouver system, **81**
   Harvard system, **82**
   Use of computer referencing packages, **84**
   Conclusion, **85**

9 Posing an evidence-based practice question: Using the PICO
   and SPICE models, **86**
   Alan Glasper and Colin Rees

   What is the PICO model?, **86**
   Examples of PICO formulated questions, 88
   What is the SPICE model?, **90**
   References, **92**

**Section 3 Developing your healthcare/evidence-based
practice dissertation, 93**

10 Managing your time wisely, **95**
    Alan Glasper and Colin Rees

    A dissertation as a frame of mind, **96**
    Conclusion, **98**
    References, **100**

11 Developing your study skills, **101**
    Alan Glasper and Colin Rees

    Knowing yourself, **103**
    Being organised, **106**

Organising things in terms of what goes where, **107**
Consolidating your ideas and activities by talking to others
about it, **107**
Reference, **107**

12 Getting the most from your supervisor, **108**
Judith Lathlean

How to get started, **108**
Agreeing a working pattern, **109**
Anticipating and preventing problems, **109**
Good planning is the essence, **109**
Supervision at a distance, **110**
Additional support, **111**
Resources, **112**

**Section 4 Preparing to use research evidence in your
dissertation, 113**

13 Understanding quantitative research, **115**
Alan Glasper and Colin Rees

Is it a quantitative study?, **115**
Why quantitative?, **117**
Types of quantitative studies, **117**
Key elements in a quantitative study, **120**
Strengths of quantitative studies, **120**
Limitations, **124**
Conclusion, **124**
References, **124**

14 Understanding qualitative research, **126**
Alan Glasper and Colin Rees

Why qualitative?, **127**
Types of qualitative studies, **128**
Key elements in a qualitative study, **129**
Strengths of qualitative studies, **131**
Limitations, **132**
Conclusion, **132**
References, **133**

Section 5 Critically appraising evidence, 135

15 Selecting and using appraisal tools: How to interrogate research papers, **137**
Alan Glasper and Colin Rees

Introduction, **137**
What is critical appraisal? What are critical appraisal tools?
   Why is critical appraisal of published research important?
   What does critical appraisal mean to nurses and other
   healthcare professionals?, **138**
What is the best critical appraisal tool to use?, **139**
Commencing your critique, **140**
Is an individual paper worth adding to the short list? Preparing your
   initial long short list, **140**
Commencing your initial read and review of an empirical
   journal paper, **141**
Points to consider about the paper(s) before using any critiquing tool, **143**
Applying a critiquing framework tool of your choice to your selected
   papers, **145**
Critiquing models, **147**
Conclusion, **156**
References, **157**

16 Critically reviewing qualitative papers using a CASP
   critiquing tool, **158**
Di Carpenter

Screening questions, **159**
The CASP qualitative questions, **160**
Data analysis, **163**
Research findings, **163**
The value of the research, **164**
Reflection, **164**
References, **165**

17 Critically reviewing quantitative papers using a CASP
   critiquing tool, **166**
Steve George

Question 1 'Did the study ask a clearly-focused question?', **167**
Question 2 'Was this a randomised controlled trial (RCT) and was it
   appropriately so?', **168**

Question 3 'Were participants appropriately allocated to intervention
and control groups?', **171**
Question 4 'Were participants, staff and study personnel 'blind' to
participants study group?', **171**
Question 5 'Were all of the participants who entered the
trial accounted for at its conclusion?', **173**
Question 6 'Were the participants in all groups followed
up and data collected in the same way?', **173**
Question 7 'Did the study have enough participants to
minimise the play of chance?', **174**
Question 8 'How are the results presented and what is the
main result?', **174**
Question 9 'How precise are these results?', **176**
Question 10 'Were all important outcomes considered so the
results can be applied?', **176**

18 Critically reviewing a journal paper using the Parahoo
model, **177**
Kader Parahoo and Irene Heuter

Introduction, **177**
Framework for appraisal, **178**
Conclusion, **186**
References, **186**

19 Critically reviewing a journal paper using the Rees model, **187**
Alan Glasper and Colin Rees

Conclusion, **192**
References, **193**

**Section 6 How evidence-based healthcare is implemented
in practice, 195**

20 Using evidence in practice, **197**
Tracey Harding, Lisa Harding and Alan Glasper

Introduction, **197**
Applying research findings to practice: using and applying
evidence in practice, **198**
Potential barriers to the implementation of change, **205**
Change management strategies, **209**
Review and evaluation of effectiveness of change, **212**

Leadership of change, **214**
Using Government policy guidance to help implement
  evidence-based practice, **216**
Can high impact nursing actions result in enhanced
  patient care?, **219**
Conclusion, **223**
References, **223**

**Section 7 Taking your dissertation further: disseminating
evidence, knowledge transfer; writing as a
professional skill, 227**

21 Publishing your dissertation: In a journal or at a conference, **229**
   John Fowler and Colin Rees

   Your dissertation is complete: what next?, **229**
   Motivation, **230**
   Conference abstract and presentation, **231**
   Writing a paper for publication, **235**
   What will you do with your dissertation?, **241**

22 Reflecting on your dissertation journey, **242**
   Wendy Wigley

   Reflection, **242**
   Frameworks for reflection, **244**
   Some final points on reflection, **248**
   References, **249**

23 Building the architecture of your dissertation, **250**
   Alan Glasper and Colin Rees

   Writing your evidence-based practice thesis, **250**
   Reference, **255**

24 Glossary of common research and statistical terms, **256**
   Colin Rees and Peter Nicholls

**Section 8 Bonus chapters (Website only)
www.wiley.com/go/glasper/nursingdissertation, 273**

25 Developing a public health evidence-based practice dissertation
   Palo Almond

26 Using historical literature
    Di Carpenter

27 Managing a learning difference
    Michelle Cowen

28 Interpreting statistics
    Peter Nicholls

29 Research governance in practice
    Vikki Yule and Martina Prude

30 Developing mechanisms to change clinical practice in the light
    of evidence: A case study
    Valerie Wilson

31 Clinical standards, audit and inspection
    Alan Glasper and Colin Rees

Index, **275**

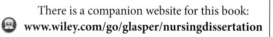

There is a companion website for this book:
www.wiley.com/go/glasper/nursingdissertation

List of Contributors

Dr Palo Almond
Head of Primary and Public Health
Anglia Ruskin University
Fulbourn, Cambridgeshire, UK

Paul Boagy
Former Senior Librarian
University of Southampton, UK

Dr Di Carpenter
Mental Health Nursing Lead Faculty of Health Sciences
University of Southampton, UK

Michelle Cowen
Principal Teaching Fellow/Faculty Lead for Disability
and Dyslexia Faculty of Health Sciences
University of Southampton, UK

Dr John Fowler
Senior Lecturer in Nursing
Sheffield Hallam University, UK

Dr Steve George
Reader in Public Health
School of Medicine
University of Southampton, UK

Dr Alan Glasper
Professor of Nursing and Top-up Degree Programme Lead
Faculty of Health Sciences
University of Southampton, UK

Lisa Harding
Lecturer/Programme Leader
University of Winchester, UK

Tracey Harding
Lecturer in Nursing Faculty of Health Sciences
University of Southampton, UK

Irene Heuter
Professor of Statistics
Columbia University
New York, NY, USA

Dr Judith Lathlean
Professor Faculty of Health Sciences
University of Southampton, UK

Dr Andrée le May
Professor of Nursing Faculty of Health Sciences
University of Southampton, UK

Dr Pat Maier
Former Deputy Vice Chancellor (Teaching and Learning)
University of Southampton, UK

Dr Peter Nicholls
Senior Statistician Faculty of Health Sciences
University of Southampton, UK

Dr Kader Parahoo
Professor of Nursing Research
University of Ulster, UK

Dr Martina Prude
Head of Ethical Governance
University of Southampton, UK

Sheila Reading
Lecturer in Nursing Faculty of Health Sciences
University of Southampton, UK

Colin Rees
MSc in Nursing Programme Manager
University of Cardiff, UK

Wendy Wigley
Lecturer Public Health
University of Southampton, UK

Dr Valerie Wilson
Director of Nursing Research & Practice Development
The Children's Hospital at Westmead
Professor of Nursing Research & Practice Development
The University of Technology Sydney
NSW, Australia

Vikki Yule
Former Research Governance Lead
Southampton University Hospitals NHS Trust, UK

Foreword

Only twenty years ago, the idea that students should be taught about the evidence that underpins clinical practice was regarded as a dangerously radical one. This book shows how great the change over the intervening period has been. During that time small communities of researchers and methodologists have created alliances with practitioners and patients around specific clinical problems. They have subjected what is known about the clinical and cost effectiveness of different treatments and modes of professional practice to rigorous tests, using primary studies, clinical trials, systematic reviews and meta-analyses. In almost every area of healthcare, the application of evidence has led to a revolution in the quality of care that patients receive.

This book is part of that revolution, and every chapter is written by practitioners with real life experience of understanding and applying evidence. Each chapter is written in a way that emphasises its application to real life problems. This is important because 'evidence' isn't an abstract problem. And it isn't just a problem for students either. Politicians, policy makers and managers all struggle with evidence, and seek ways to make it meaningful to their own situations. Sometimes this means that evidence isn't always what it seems. My own research has shown how clinical trials of new health technologies are hard for their sponsors to fathom (May, 2006), and how policy makers seek quite different kinds of evidence for their effectiveness that sometimes fit poorly with wider conceptions of robustness and rigour but very well with the interests and goals of organisations (May, 2007).

So, evidence is important because it offers a rational basis for the allocation of healthcare resources and the provision of patient care. But what is and isn't evidence isn't just a problem of method. Underpinning that problem is a deeper one, alluded to in almost every chapter in the book – but particularly in Diane Carpenter's chapter on historical methods and evidence – which is that what counts as evidence is sometimes contingent on time and place.

If evidence is important because it offers a rational basis for practice, it's worth remembering that much of what we see practiced every day in hospitals and clinics has no evidence base. The challenge for a new generation of students is to change that. This book will start to give you the tools to achieve that.

Carl May
Professor of Healthcare Innovation
Faculty of Health Sciences
University of Southampton

May, C. (2006) Mobilizing modern facts: Health Technology Assessment and the politics of evidence. *Sociology of Health & Illness*, **28**, 513–532.

May, C. (2007) The clinical encounter and the problem of context. *Sociology*, **41**, 29–45.

Preface

This book provides the reader with a clear knowledge of the fundamental steps needed to write an evidence-based practice healthcare dissertation at honours degree and master's levels.

It aims to bring together key ideas and concepts related to evidence-based practice and research use pertinent to the production of a dissertation. Using practical examples, the book will demonstrate the way in which all the components of evidence-based healthcare, such as research use skills, standard setting, legal and ethical frameworks, audit and benchmarking, are drawn together for the purpose of a dissertation.

Primary target

The main audience for this book is nurses and other healthcare professionals who are required to complete an evidence-based practice dissertation as part fulfilment of an honours or master's degree.

Secondary target

This guide to evidence-based practice will also be used by pre-registration healthcare undergraduates and qualified staff who require this knowledge for their day-to-day clinical activities.

Style of the book

The book is written using a very clear and engaging scenario style. This has been used to provide a logical structure and progression to the ideas embodied within the text that readers will find relevant to their dissertation work.

We are confident that this book will provide you, the reader, with a clear knowledge of the fundamental aspects of evidence-based practice needed to provide accurate and high quality care within current healthcare systems.

About the companion website

There is a companion website available for this book at
www.wiley.com/go/glasper/nursingdissertation

On the site you will find:
- Seven bonus chapters
- Summary of each chapter in the accompanying book
- A range of tools and frameworks
- Sample documents to assist you writing your dissertation
- Useful reference links
- Reference lists for each chapter

The website is signposted throughout the book. Look out for this icon.

Acknowledgements

The author of this book are grateful to Lisa Lewis for permitting the inclusion of her dissertation on the companion website.

Thanks also to Dr Peter Carter, Chief Executive of the RCN for giving permission for the complete RCN document to be hosted on the website and to Professor Dame Christine Beasley (now former chief Nursing Officer for England) for being so supportive of the book and for access to the essential collection.

The scenarios

Sue is a 40-year-old senior staff nurse who works in an elderly care unit of a large tertiary teaching hospital. She entered nursing late after having a family and completed her enhanced diploma in adult nursing four years earlier. Her ward manager has sponsored her to undertake a 'top-up degree' programme at her local university. The programme she has enrolled on is specially designed to allow enhanced/advanced diplomate holders to progress towards gaining an honours degree classification. In essence, the course entails attending a number of taught study days, where she will learn about the nuts and bolts of understanding evidence-based practice. The assessment, which if successfully completed, will confer upon her a degree classification that is based on the submission of a 10 000 word dissertation. Sue has not opened a text book for nearly five years and although she tries to keep up to date by reading a nursing journal which her ward subscribes to she is full of trepidation about the course she has enrolled on.

Her good friend and neighbour, Sam, aged 31, works in the local children's hospital as a ward manager. He is already a graduate, having completed a degree in children's nursing some 10 years ago. Sam, likewise, has been out of the studying habit for many years. He is now seeking to become a clinical nurse specialist and has been fortunate to receive funding from his hospital to undertake an MSc in Nursing at the same university as Sue. Sam has a 'learning difference' and is Dyslexic. The dissertation element of the MSc programme is similar to the undergraduate dissertation; it is in the format of a critical review of the evidence base for practice but this time is 20 000 words in length. Sam is equally worried about completing the dissertation element of the course.

Scenario 1 – Starting the dissertation journey

Sue and Sam are facing the next challenge in their academic journey – the writing and completion of a dissertation. There is something about the dissertation that unsettles the two friends, which might be related to the size of the assignment or the freedom in choosing a project title. In reality, the dissertation gives them great freedom to choose what excites them as professionals working in clinical domains, but there are some principles that each will have to follow in developing their ideas.

Scenario 2 – Sourcing and accessing evidence for your disseration

Sue asks Sam for advice. She has some ideal 'evidence' for her dissertation but it is from a 'Sunday Supplement Magazine'; does this count as evidence, she asks? Sam tells her about the work of Professor Andrée le May.

Scenario 3 – Identifying a topic for your dissertation, setting the scene

Sam has selected a likely topic for his dissertation and wants to explore the lived experiences of families with a child with a chronic illness, but wants to ensure that it is suitable for a dissertation. He talks to Sue about her choice, which is the use of larvae therapy for wound healing in older women with varicose leg ulcers (NB: to provide variety and relevance within the book, some of the chapters use different dissertation topics to illustrate key points).

Scenario 4 – Preparing to use research evidence in your dissertation

At this point Sam is looking for qualitative studies to use in his dissertation and Sue is looking for Randomised Controlled Trials that will help her answer her dissertation question. One of Sue's friends wants to examine historical literature.

Scenario 5 – Critically appraising evidence

Having collected some relevant research articles, both Sue and Sam are faced with selecting an appropriate critical appraisal tool to evaluate their selected papers. Sam has been advised to use Parahoo's critiquing approach.

Scenario 6 – How evidence-based healthcare is implemented in practice

Over coffee Sam tells Sue that he has a great lead for his dissertation. He has found a range of papers on work done in Sydney Children's Hospital, where they have had success in implementing evidence-based practice. Additionally, Sue has read some of Professor Peter Callery's work.

Scenario 7 – Clinical standards, audit and inspection

Sue's clinical area is being audited by the English healthcare watch dog, The Care Quality Commission.

Scenario 8 – Taking your dissertation further: disseminating evidence, knowledge transfer; writing as a professional skill

Sam has been asked to present a poster based on his dissertation for a forth-coming hospital conference. Sue wants to write a paper for publication in a well-known national nursing journal.

Section 1 **Starting your dissertation journey**

Sue is a 40-year-old senior staff nurse who works in an elderly care unit of a large tertiary teaching hospital. She entered nursing late after having a family and completed her enhanced diploma in adult nursing four years earlier. Her ward manager has sponsored her to undertake a 'top-up degree' programme at her local university. The programme she has enrolled on is specially designed to allow enhanced/advanced diplomate holders to progress towards gaining an honours degree classification. In essence, the course entails attending a number of taught study days, where she will learn about the nuts and bolts of understanding evidence-based practice. The assessment, which if successfully completed, will confer upon her a degree classification that is based on the submission of a 10 000 word dissertation. Sue has not opened a text book for nearly five years and although she tries to keep up to date by reading a nursing journal which her ward subscribes to she is full of trepidation about the course she has enrolled on.

Her good friend and neighbour, Sam, aged 31, works in the local children's hospital as a ward manager. He is already a graduate, having completed a degree in children's nursing some 10 years ago. Sam, likewise, has been out of the studying habit for many years. He is now seeking to become a clinical nurse specialist and has been fortunate to receive funding from his hospital to undertake an MSc in Nursing at the same university as Sue. Sam has a 'learning difference' and is Dyslexic. The dissertation element of the MSc programme is similar to the undergraduate dissertation; it is in the format of a critical review of the evidence base for practice but this time is 20 000 words in length. Sam is equally worried about completing the dissertation element of the course.

Sue and Sam are facing the next challenge in their academic journey – the writing and completion of a dissertation. There is something about the dissertation that unsettles the two friends, which might be related to the size of the assignment or the freedom in choosing a project title. In reality, the dissertation gives them great freedom to choose what excites them as professionals working in clinical domains, but there are some principles that each will have to follow in developing their ideas.

Chapter 1 **Starting your dissertation journey**

Sheila Reading
University of Southampton, UK

What are dissertations?

There are many different types of student academic assignments that are referred to as dissertations. Normally a dissertation is a major piece of independent research-based study undertaken towards the end of a healthcare programme. The nature of dissertations varies both across academic disciplines and Higher Education Institutions (HEIs) in terms of length, focus and timing. Healthcare professionals are often required to submit an evidence-based practice dissertation as part of their undergraduate or postgraduate programme. A dissertation is often viewed as the culmination of a programme of learning which helps consolidate the student's knowledge, skills and understanding of the research base of the discipline.

Scenario

Sue, a senior staff nurse, has an Advanced Diploma in Nursing and is aware of the move to an all graduate profession for new applicants to nursing. This has prompted her to embark on a 'top-up degree' programme at a nearby university to enable her to achieve graduate status. To meet the programme requirements she will need to complete a 10 000 word evidence-based practice dissertation.

Her friend Sam, who is a ward manager, graduated with a Bachelor in Nursing degree ten years earlier and now wants to study for an MSc in Nursing. For a Master's evidence-based practice dissertation, he will have to write a thesis of 20 000 words in length.

Both are chatting together about the task ahead and their feelings about having to complete such lengthy assignments. Neither is yet completely certain what subject to focus on for their dissertation and both are anxious to begin to understand what will be expected of them. The word length required is perceived to be arduous and daunting.

How to Write Your Nursing Dissertation, First Edition. Alan Glasper and Colin Rees.
© 2013 John Wiley & Sons, Ltd. Published 2013 by John Wiley & Sons, Ltd.

> SUE: 'Why do we have to write such a long dissertation?'
>
> SAM: 'That is a good question Sue. We should first explore what evidence-based practice dissertation is so we can understand why it is a significant aspect of our degree programmes and what we need to achieve. This article I have been reading indicates some key aspects of a dissertation.'

First, the learner determines the focus and direction of the work. Second, this work is carried out on an individual basis – although usually with some tutor support and direction provided. Third, there is typically a substantial research component to the project requiring analysis of existing/secondary data. Finally, learners will have a more prolonged engagement with the chosen subject than is the case with 'standard' coursework assignments, such as essays or reports, with the work consequently expected to be more 'in depth'.

(Todd, Bannister and Clegg, 2004:335)

Activity

Before reading further it will be helpful for you to consider what you think an evidence-based practice dissertation is and what you are expected to do.

Talk to others who have completed a dissertation and seek out information from the university where you will study. Try to read sample dissertations. The university where you are studying will normally have a number of examples in its library for you to examine. (The website that accompanies this book hosts a sample top-up degree dissertation. Go to www.wiley.com/go/glasper/nursingdissertation)

Aim to be clear about what is expected of you for your dissertation work.

Dissertations are accepted as a highly valued part of both undergraduate and Master's degrees. The UK Quality Assurance Agency (QAA) benchmark statements for healthcare programmes substantiate the importance of dissertations. In particular, one of the expectations of the QAA (2001) is that the healthcare professional can contribute to the development and dissemination of evidence-based practice within professional contexts. This is what studying for an evidence-based practice dissertation aspires to achieve for the individual student.

The Royal College of Nursing (RCN, 2011) has published its strategy to help nurses improve the use of evidence in practice; it helps them to source information, interpret, synthesise and communicate it. (A full PDF copy of this valuable resource is available from the companion website at www.wiley.com/go/glasper/nursingdissertation.)

Healthcare practitioners need to be able to ask questions about practice, access healthcare research and evidence and report the key ideas and findings

> **Activity**
>
> Access the companion website of this book and read Royal College of Nursing publication, *Finding, using and managing information. Nursing, midwifery, health and social care information literacy competencies* (RCN, 2011).

effectively and accurately to others. Preparing a dissertation encourages practitioners to become more familiar with relevant theoretical knowledge and literature, which promotes a better understanding of the practice topic being explored.

Boud and Costley (2007:119) highlight that the activities undertaken for dissertations, a major aspect of degree studies, relate to both the learning needs of the student, education values and the world of work. Undertaking a dissertation is an indication of the ability of students to manage their own learning (Stephenson, 1998), communicate and make decisions.

The dissertation demonstrates a link between research, personal learning and professional practice. It is as much about the learning gained during the process as the presentation of the final product – the bound dissertation. Production of an evidence-based dissertation is the primary means to achieving an honours degree, or a Master's degree.

> **Scenario**
>
> Sue is wondering about the difference between the undergraduate dissertation she will have to complete, compared with that which Sam will complete at Master's level.
>
> SAM: 'I guess it is more than just a difference in word length! But let's think about this.'

Normally, an undergraduate dissertation will be based on a critique of a small selection of evidence and be applied to one focused aspect of the student's practice. It will provide insight and hands-on experience of the process of engaging in evidence-based practice and should inform individual or local professional clinical practice.

The requirement of a Master's programme is that the evidence-based dissertation demonstrates how the student has 'mastered' a core aspect of healthcare practice and the related research knowledge and discipline-related content. There is a *qualitative* difference between the master's dissertation and the undergraduate dissertation as well as the *quantitive* difference recognised by the word allowance. This normally relates to the depth, breadth and analysis demonstrated in the written work. A Master's dissertation will systematically critique a greater amount of evidence from a range of different sources, demonstrating a significant appreciation of underlying issues and application and impact of the findings for the wider practice context.

Undergraduate evidence-based practice dissertations tend to focus on 'what' and 'where' questions related to practice, while Master's level work will move on to asking more analytical questions which focus on the 'how' and 'why' of practice.

QAA subject benchmark statements provide a means of describing standards for the award of qualifications at a given level. The capabilities and attributes of those who undertake dissertations for particular qualifications should demonstrate the appropriate level of study. This is always indicated in the programme dissertation assignment guidelines and the learning outcomes made available to students. More detail on this can be found in Chapter 2.

Tip: As well as significant differences in word length and the scope and depth of analysis required, the period available to complete and the expected hours of self-directed study between an undergraduate and postgraduate masters dissertation will differ. Make sure you have explored in detail the dissertation requirements of your programme and use them to help you organise and plan for the task ahead.

What are the features of a degree education?

Scenario

Sam and Sue are discussing what a degree education offers.

SAM: I think I need to be clear about why I am planning to undertake academic study again and what a master's degree will offer me personally and professionally in terms of development. I want to become a clinical nurse specialist.

SUE: I agree. I am already an experienced staff nurse with confidence in my skills but I do want to become a graduate like other health care professionals we work with. I am hoping to learn more about my practice and how to make best decisions for my practice and for patient care.

SAM: I think we both want to develop professionally and respond to new challenges, clinically and academically, as well as enhancing our knowledge and skills to further extend our expertise in our field of practice. Is this the basis of undergraduate and postgraduate education?

The goal of graduate education as outlined by the Nursing and Midwifery Council (NMC, 2010) standards is to equip nurses with the knowledge, skills and behaviours to respond to changing needs and expectations in healthcare. A key requirement is that graduate nurse's make person-centred, evidence-based judgements and decisions in practice. Graduate education promotes an evidence-based approach to delivering appropriate healthcare in an effective way to individuals (Pearson and Craig, 2002).

Increasingly, degree programmes are aligned with the achievement of defined 'graduate attributes'. Many HEIs have identified their own specific graduate attributes. These usually focus on skills which are valuable for, and transferable to, work-based contexts. Graduate attributes support learners in meeting the needs of a complex, challenging and constantly changing environment of employment. They include more than just the academic or professional skills of the discipline and demonstrate skills needed to be independent, autonomous and lifelong learners, which are viewed as important characteristics of being a graduate. Graduate attributes include personal qualities, skills and knowledge gained as a result of engaging in study. They include qualities such as adopting academic approaches to thinking which demonstrate openness to new ways of responding to unfamiliar situations and challenges with intellectual curiosity.

In addition to developing skills in information retrieval and critiquing research evidence, completing a degree equips individuals with highly prized transferable skills, such as problem solving, project management and report writing, which can significantly enhance professional communication and practice. In a study to elucidate research related graduate attributes, Laidlaw, Guild and Struthers (2009) found evidence to support the case for dissertations helping achieve both clinical and research related graduate attributes for medical undergraduates. The attributes included: an inquiring mind, core knowledge, critical appraisal, understanding the evidence base for professional practice, understanding ethics and governance, and an ability to communicate. Each of these graduate attributes could be argued as being relevant for other healthcare professionals.

Completing an honours degree is often a precursor to further academic study, such as a postgraduate Masters or doctoral studies. A Master's dissertation will build on previous knowledge gained at undergraduate level and develop new understandings and a greater breadth depth of learning. Each stage is part of a progressive development of research knowledge and skills. This may be part of developing a Clinical Academic Career pathway which integrates research and education to improve the use of research, and other evidence, in clinical practice (UKCRC, 2007).

> **Activity**
>
> Sam and Sue know why they want to undertake a degree and at what level.
>   Try and think of all the reasons why you want to and write a list. Prioritise the items and write a short summary statement to refer back to later.

Features of a dissertation

A dissertation is an extended and substantial piece of work carried out independently. It is common to have a link with a group of peers who are also completing a dissertation with the same submission date and to have a link with a member of the university staff who will supervise and offer academic support. The dissertation is quite different from other assignments in terms of its depth and the length of time engaged with it. While it may be divided into sections or chapters, it needs to demonstrate a coherent and well-structured format which poses a question that is then addressed and answered in relation to a specific practice issue.

The initial choice of topic selected can increase the personal and professional depth of understanding on the subject. Very often the breadth of knowledge may be extended into unexpected areas. For example, a recent dissertation which focused on enhancing the care of people with long term conditions in one NHS Trust led the student to an exploration of concepts of clinical leadership, while another student, also focusing on long term conditions, explored the evidence for promoting approaches to self-care.

Whatever topic is chosen, it is important to remember that sustained motivation to undertake a dissertation requires considerable enthusiasm for both the subject and the process over an extended period.

> **Scenario**
>
> For Sue and Sam, who are both experienced practitioners, the dissertations which they undertake will enable them to select subjects or topics that relate directly to their own practice locations. This enables them to draw on their experience and knowledge of health care practice and patient care and to build on that expertise.

The key features of a dissertation include:
- Title
- Well framed question
- Clear aims and objectives
- Search strategy for best evidence
- Critical appraisal of research or other best evidence
- Discussion of results and implication for practice.

This will all have to be written-up in a readable style, communicating the relevant information and presented in an understandable format according to regulations, and submitted on time.

Undertaking a dissertation will be both challenging and rewarding. In a study examining the student dissertation experience, Harrison and Whalley (2008) found that common difficulties encountered included: deciding on a topic for study, time management, writing up a large dissertation and dealing with stress.

Presenting the result of a study into student's thoughts of their dissertation experience, Harrison and Whalley (2008:408) provide examples which highlight some of the perceived tensions. The following are examples:

- 'Felt that I learned as much about myself as I did about the topic.'
- 'There is no doubting completing my dissertation was one of the most stressful times of my life but at the same time the most rewarding.'
- 'I enjoyed having the chance to show what I am capable of. I found it very stressful at times, but achieved huge sense of satisfaction when over.'

Producing a dissertation demonstrates and communicates that you have consolidated a range of skills, including intellectual, professional, information seeking, critical analysis and synthesis of knowledge.

Planning your dissertation – essential considerations

A brief outline on how dissertations are planned is given here; more details are given in Chapter 2.

Planning your available time

Some students find the use of Gantt charts helpful (Table 1.1).

Table 1.1 Example of a Gantt chart.

	Oct	Nov	Dec	Jan	Feb	Mar	Apr	May	Jun
Select topic	——→								
Search and select evidence	———————————→								
Critically appraise evidence				———————————→					
Write up chapters	———————————————————————→								
Conclusions Discussions					———————————————→				

It is important to be clear about how much time to allocate to each step of the process. Several stages may be undertaken at a time and undertaking a dissertation is not always a linear process.

It is sensible to remember that things do not always run according to plan. Life events can interfere and mean that work is delayed. It makes sense to build in time for some slippage to prevent a last minute panic in meeting the deadline for submission of the dissertation. Do allow time for making final revisions and checking for spelling or other errors.

Begin writing early – produce drafts to show others and get feedback

While the list of things to do indicated above gives an outline of the structure for the written dissertation, careful thought is need about how best to present the final coherent dissertation. Reading other dissertations written by students who have completed similar programmes is always a good resource for considering how to frame your headings, sections and chapters. However, each dissertation is unique and support from a supervisor in interpreting the assignment guidelines to apply to your own evidence based dissertation is always essential.

For example, at times it can be difficult to know where to end the results section and begin the conclusions. It is important to weave all the sections together into the whole, which is the final written dissertation.

It is important to avoid writing too descriptively. Remember you need to adopt an academic approach, demonstrating your ability to think critically and analytically and to synthesise conclusions from all the information you have gathered.

Get support from others

Enlist family and friends to encourage you in keeping on task. Work with peers on the programme who are going through the same experience as you; email them or meet informally to discuss aspects of each other's work and for mutual support. Take opportunities offered to present your ideas to the programme group or your academic supervisor in order to get supportive feedback. Some universities have special sections of their electronic learning platforms (e.g. Backboard) which feature student chat-rooms where information can be exchanged.

Adopt the help of 'critical readers', not necessarily those familiar with your topic, or even with healthcare, who can proofread your writing and check if the structure of your dissertation is coherent and makes sense.

Finally back up everything you save on your computer!

Tip: Buy several (minimum four megabytes) data/memory sticks/USB flash drives to store copies of your work.

Create a folder entitled my dissertation with subfolders for each individual chapter.

Completing your dissertation and gaining a good classification

Because the dissertation at undergraduate or postgraduate level makes a significant contribution in terms of credits gained and to the student's final classification, it is often an important priority for students to gain a good result.

Scenario

Sue and Sam are wondering what makes an outstanding dissertation and how they can achieve the best possible marks.

SUE: What do you think the markers will be looking for Sam?

SAM: Well, I think they will want to see more than five 2000 word essays, Sue. At the moment you seem to have five chapters written at separate times. It will need to be coherent and feature only relevant information.

SUE: I guess I need to make the chapters flow into each other. The difficulty is knowing what to leave out. I seem to be well over the word limit.

SAM: Well, we could read each other's work and offer some feedback, then meet with our supervisors and check if we are doing as well as we hope. At the moment I seem to be writing too descriptively.

🖥   The companion website at www.wiley.com/go/glasper/nursingdissertation hosts a very good example of an undergraduate dissertation.

Make sure you meet the deadlines for submitting the final dissertation for marking and that you are not rushed towards the end. Being short of time can lead to you taking short cuts and, potentially, reduce the time available to complete your writing to the required standard. Remember, time is needed to refine drafts, ensure accurate reference lists, and check for typographical and other errors related to the general presentation before the dissertation is to be bound. Be clear about the written style (font and spacing) and final presentation format required by your university and degree programme.

To achieve a good grade you will need to look at the module assignment guidelines, learning outcomes and marking criteria (Table 1.2). Universities normally explain the basis on which student dissertations are assessed in order to guide student learning and, importantly, to ensure work is marked fairly and consistently. It is very important that as a student you are familiar with the dissertation requirements and marking guidance. Often a module handbook is produced by the university that will give details of the dissertation expectations and the explicit marking criteria by which they will be assessed. This can be discussed with your supervisor at an early stage and as you complete written sections or chapters. Part of your own learning is to

Table 1.2 Example of possible evidence-based dissertation marking criteria.

Category	Relative importance (%)
Presentation (structure, language, referencing)	8
Abstract (accuracy, relevance and clarity)	2
Introduction (background to project, issues to be addressed, background reading, framing of the question)	20
Identification and selection of best evidence (retrieval of evidence, search strategy and terms, rationale for criteria to select or reject evidence, audit trail)	20
Critical appraisal of evidence (rationale for selection of critiquing framework/tool, judgement of evidence, rigour, addresses the question, research understanding)	25
Conclusions and implications for practice (conclusions well drawn from selected evidence, skills of analysis and evaluation, relevance to practice, application to practice)	15
Discussion and plan for implementation	10

develop your skills in self-assessment so that you can recognise the standard of work which you are capable of and need to aim for to ensure the desired grade.

For Sue and Sam, who are both experienced practitioners, the dissertations which they undertake will enable them to select subjects or topics that relate directly to their own practice environments. This enables them to draw on their experience and knowledge of healthcare practice and patient care and to build on that expertise.

References

Boud, D. and Costley, C. (2007) From project supervision to advising: new conceptions of the practice. *Innovations in Education and Teaching International*, **44** (2), 119–130.

Harrison, M.E. and Whalley, B. (2008) Undertaking a dissertation form start to finish: the process and product. *Journal of Geography in Higher Education*, **32** (3), 401–418.

Laidlaw, A., Guild, S. and Struthers, J. (2009) Graduate attributes in the disciplines of medicine, dentistry and veterinary medicine: a survey of expert opinions. *BMC Medical Education*, **9** (28). doi:10.1186/1472-6920-9-28.

NMC (2010) Standards of proficiency for pre-registration nursing education 2004 (updated 2010). Nursing and Midwifery Council, London.

Pearson, M. and Craig, J.V. (2002) Evidence based practice in nursing. In: Craig, J.V. and Smyth, R.L., *The evidence-based practice manual for nurses*, 209–233. Churchill Livingstone, London.

QAA (2001) Subject benchmarks for health care professionals –Nursing. Quality Assurance Agency (QAA) for Higher Education, Gloucester.

RCN (2011) Finding, using and managing information. Nursing, midwifery, health and social care information literacy competencies. The Royal College of Nursing, London.

Stephenson, J. (1998) Supporting student autonomy in learning. In: Stephenson, J. and Yorke, M. (eds), *Capability and quality in higher education*, pp. 129–141. Kogan Page, London.

Todd, M., Bannister, P. and Clegg, S. (2004) Independent inquiry and the undergraduate dissertation: perceptions and experiences of social science students. *Assessment and Education in Higher Education*, **29** (3), 335–355.

UKCRC (2007) Report of the UKCRC Subcommittee for Nurses in Clinical Research (Workforce). UK Clinical Research Collaboration (UKCRC), London.

Further reading

Bell, J. (2005) 4th Edition *Doing your research project: A Guide for first time researchers in education, health and social sciences*. Open University Press, Maidenhead.

Greetham, B. (2009) *How to write your undergraduate dissertation*. Palgrave study skills, Palgrave Macmillan, Basingstoke.

O'Loughlin, E.F.M. (2011) How to create a basic Gantt Chart in Microsoft Excel 2010. http://www.youtube.com/watch?v=sA67g6zaKOE&noredirect=1 (accessed 15 May 2012).

Walliman, N. and Appleton, J. (2009) *Your Undergraduate Dissertation in Health and Social Care*. Sage Publications, London.

For further resources for this chapter visit the companion website at
www.wiley.com/go/glasper/nursingdissertation

Chapter 2 Introduction to writing your evidence-based practice dissertation

Alan Glasper[1] and Colin Rees[2]
[1]*University of Southampton, UK*
[2]*University of Cardiff, UK*

Scenario

Sue and Sam are facing the next challenge in their academic journey – the writing and completion of a dissertation. There is something about the dissertation that unsettles the two friends, which might be related to the size of the assignment or the freedom in choosing a project title. In reality, the dissertation gives them great freedom to choose what excites them as professionals working in clinical domains, but there are some principles that each will have to follow in developing their ideas.

Most healthcare students undertaking an undergraduate or postgraduate course have to submit a dissertation as part of the assessment process. The learning outcomes of the dissertation may differ but the basic architecture remains the same.

Sample guidelines for students undertaking an undergraduate healthcare dissertation

All students need to read carefully the particular university assessment guidelines for whichever course they are undertaking. The dissertation usually takes the form of an evidence-based practice project that focuses in-depth on a clinical/practice focused issue. Students normally identify an issue arising from their own practice area, and will further develop this into a question to guide the dissertation.

Typical dissertations will include the following sections:
- Introduction and rationale for selection of the topic area.

How to Write Your Nursing Dissertation, First Edition. Alan Glasper and Colin Rees.
© 2013 John Wiley & Sons, Ltd. Published 2013 by John Wiley & Sons, Ltd.

- Review of literature relating to the subject area leading to the generation of the research question or recommendations for practice.
- Strategy for collection of evidence, including database search range/terminology.
- Critical appraisal and evaluation of evidence relating to the topic.
- Analysis of the findings.
- Discussion and synthesis of the extent to which the evidence reviewed answers the research question.
- Critical discussion on implementation of the project findings to practice, incorporating consideration of the culture of the organisation, leadership styles and change management strategies best suited to achieve this.

Typical learning outcomes for an undergraduate evidence-based practice dissertation

1 Demonstrate the ability to systematically search and critically appraise evidence, including literature/primary research/systematic reviews/clinical guidelines using an appropriate critical appraisal framework(s).
2 Critically analyse practice and identify a clinical issue for exploration.
3 Demonstrate a critical awareness and knowledge of research methodology.
4 Reflect on the breadth of evidence that underpins practice.
5 Derive solutions to problems based on the collection, interrogation and interpretation of information and data obtained from a variety of sources, and draw on established analytical techniques in the broad field of health and social care.
6 Demonstrate self-reflection and an understanding of the limitations of the key concepts of the underpinning disciplines.
7 Demonstrate confidence in understanding, manipulating, interpreting and presenting numerical narrative data.
8 Demonstrate an understanding of the role of the student and supervisor.
9 Identify a question for an evidence-based practice project to inform a proposal and dissertation.
10 Consider ways in which styles of leadership and organisational culture impact on effective care delivery within a range of practice arenas.
11 Critically discuss the barriers and behaviours which may undermine the achievement of excellent practice.
12 Critically appraise the barriers and opportunities that will impinge on evidence-based practice within clinical care, management, education and research.

13   Consider ways in which barriers to evidence-based practice could be reduced.
14   Critically evaluate the process by which evidence can be disseminated.
15   Gather and evaluate evidence and information from a wide range of sources: to think logically, systematically and conceptually; to draw reasoned conclusions or to reach sustainable judgements, and to apply these to practice.

The dissertation

For many students, the idea of producing a 10 000 (undergraduate) word or 20 000 (postgraduate Master's course) word dissertation is a daunting one, despite this figure rising up to 80 000 words for a PhD.

However, it need not be overwhelming. This chapter has been designed to help you understand what is required as you embark on this personal academic journey. It is important to set yourself achievable and manageable target dates for each stage of your dissertation journey (and try to keep to them!). Many universities will allocate you an educational supervisor who will guide and support you through the process.

Selecting a topic area

Many of you will have an idea of the topic you wish to explore in your dissertation and will pose of frame an evidence based question usually related to your own sphere of practice. Once you have framed a question you will search the scholarly literature for evidence to allow you to answer your question. This will be achieved through a comprehensive process we describe in this book involving a range of reputable databases. Normally you can trust your own university or hospital librarian to help you with this task. Some universities will ask you to submit a 1500-word proposal prior to the commencement of your dissertation. This may be formative (no grade allocated) or summative (where a mark is given and this contributes to the total mark awarded for the dissertation). The proposal will require a comprehensive outline of the proposed evidence-based practice project and will provide the opportunity for feedback and consideration prior to commencing the the dissertation.

Supervision

Most universities have a code of conduct relating to supervision (where provided) and it is normally the responsibility of the student to consult their supervisor to discuss any problems and to seek guidance on aspects of the work The amount of supervision time students are entitled to also varies depending upon the level of the course being undertaken, more for a PhD and less for an undergraduate course.

Educational supervision will usually be provided by a member of the academic team who either has experience in the area of the student's project or of the methodology to be used. A supervisor should meet the following criteria:

1 Evidence of previous research work and experience.
2 Ideally have appropriate background in the area of the project or the methodology used in the student's project.

Submission deadline

It is the student's responsibility to complete and submit the dissertation by the deadline stipulated by the individual university. This is usually an academic year. All students in university settings will have access to processes to request mitigation or special consideration. All students should read the relevant policy in their own university student handbook.

Guidelines for students undertaking an undergraduate evidence-based practice dissertation

Although these will vary from university to university, the schedule below is typical:

1 Students are required to submit a dissertation of 10 000 words, excluding diagrams, appendices, references and bibliography.
2 Two typewritten copies must be submitted. The dissertation must be typed on one side only with double spacing throughout and a margin of one inch on each side (A4 white paper). Two self-bound copies must be presented, one of which will be returned to the student. (NB: Some universities allow submission electronically via email or compact disc.)
Binding: Some universities insist that dissertations are bound. This is usually soft binding and should be preferably undertaken by a university or college bindery or an appropriate shop.
3 Typical dissertations are set out as follows:
- Title page containing:
  Name of University, Year and Faculty or School
  Full name and number of student
  Title of course
  Title of the dissertation
- Contents page listing:
  Abstract
  Acknowledgements

    Introduction
    Literature review
    Method
    Results
    Discussion of results
    Conclusions and recommendations for practice
    References (using the Modified Harvard system)
    List of tables/figures
    Glossary of terms or abbreviations
    Appendices

4   All pages must be numbered centrally at the foot of each page.
5   Presentation is important; poor or hurried proofreading will affect the quality of the dissertation. Remember to use grammar and spell-check.
6   A signed statement of originality and authorship is usually required; this may include the word count for the work. Usually, everything before the first page of the introduction is not included in the word count; the references and appendices are, similarly, not included in the word count, but do check for local variations. You will be guided locally as to where this statement sheet should be placed and if it is required to be 'bound' into the dissertation.

A frequent concern is how long each section should be. This is not easy to answer, as it will depend on available information for the sections and what is required in your educational institution. However, Table 2.1 below gives some indication of typical sections and approximate word counts.

Typical postgraduate evidence-based practice dissertation module learning outcomes

1   Demonstrate initiative, originality and justification for the construction of an original question/focus relevant to your practice/workplace, and within the wider context of health and social care.
2   Conduct an effective systematic search in relation to the question/focus that has been developed and critically appraise and evaluate the identified literature.
3   Demonstrating a comprehensive knowledge based of the different types of evidence, the research paradigms and approaches, and the ability to critically evaluate their relevance and contribution to your health and social care setting.
4   Critically analyse the relevance of any ethical and/or governance implications that may arise during the course of your enquiry.

Table 2.1   Sections, their purpose and approximate word counts (Master's Level) healthcare dissertation A.

Section title	Reason for inclusion	Aproximate word count	Evidence-based process
Abstract	Provide a succinct summary of dissertation. Usually written as a one single-spaced paragraph.	300–500	
Introduction/ Background	Orientates the reader to the practice-focussed issue: states origin of the study (personal/ professional influences); why the area invites investigation. The question is presented clarifying the explicit link to the identified clinical area of enquiry.	1500–2000	Generating the evidence
Selection and identification of the evidence	Presents the search strategy and database, including the search terms used, to illustrate depth and breadth of search. Clarifies rationale for choice of criteria used to select and reject evidence for critical appraisal.	1500–2000	Selecting the evidence
Critical appraisal of selected evidence	Identifies evidence that is relevant to the practice-related question and critically appraises this evidence through the use of a critiquing tool. Applies the selected evidence to the question set.	3000	Appraising the evidence
Conclusion and implications	Offers conclusions which address the question and which are drawn from the presented argument. Reviews how far the evidence answers the question.	1500	Determining the worth of the evidence
Plan for implementation	Offers an outline plan for implementation and dissemination. Critical discussion should demonstrate consideration of influencing factors such as the culture of the organisation, leadership styles and change management strategies best suited to achieve the plan.	1500	Implementing the evidence

5 Synthesise the evidence to address the original questions/focus and any associated issues significant to the chosen topic.

6 Demonstrate initiative in interpretation of the findings taking into account limitations and challenges of the implementation of evidence-based practice.

7 Justify the conclusions and recommendations based on insightful, comprehensive, realistic, well-reasoned arguments.

8 Demonstrate an extensive range of concepts and current research or professional issues in the chosen area of enquiry and demonstrate the ability to illustrate your unique project decision trail through the production of a coherent, logical, reflective and comprehensive report of the process, outcomes and implications of your enquiry.

9 Synthesise an innovative dissemination strategy to best influence evidence-based practice in your speciality.

Table 2.2   Guideline for sections within the dissertation.

Section	Guideline
Title page	This should detail the University, School, Award, Candidate's name and dissertation title (not included in the word count).
Abstract	This should be a concise and precise summary of the entire dissertation. It is usually presented as one single spaced paragraph. A structured abstract is recommended but should be appropriate to the nature of the project (not included in the word count).
Acknowledgements	This page is optional (not included in the word count).
Contents	This should be detailed and accurate, covering all chapters, tables, figure and appendices (not included in the word count).
Chapter 1: Introduction	This should provide comprehensive information on the topic, the rationale for its selection, its context in terms of your practice and the wider agenda for evidence-based practice in health and social care. Arising from this introduction should come the development of the aim, often in the form of the original research or practice question(s).
Chapter 2: Literature Review	This chapter details the systematic literature search strategy for the generation of data/evidence together with details of methods of appraisal. This may include any refining of the question(s), the results of the search activity and the selection of the key papers. There should be a clear decision-making trail through this chapter. It may be separate from or integrated within the following main section of the literature review chapter.

Section	Guideline
Chapter 3: Critical appraisal and synthesis of data/evidence	This chapter should demonstrate an advanced ability to critically appraise and synthesise the evidence. An excellent knowledge of the relevant research paradigms, approaches and methods that are appropriate to the selected evidence and the topic should be presented. It is expected that you will be able to critically discuss the paradigms/ approaches and offer a balanced exploration of the relative merits of each to practice and the selected topic. Ethical issues must be considered appropriately. There should be a thematic and integrated approach throughout, with clear practice / professional awareness. There should be a clear decision making trail through this chapter leading to judgements on the quality of the evidence and, hence, what evidence can be discussed in relation to promoting evidence-based practice.
Chapter 4: Discussion (Analysis of findings in context of wider literature and practice)	In addition to a discussion of findings in relation to the research/practice question(s), there should be original and creative recommendations for changing practice. Take into consideration the context of the practice setting, the current national and local health and social care agenda as well as the philosophy of evidence-based practice. You should explore where further development is needed to achieve evidence-based practice.
Chapter 5: Dissemination strategy	The dissemination strategy will need to identify an extensive range of approaches, justified with relevant theory, for presenting a clear message and to communicate effectively your evidence-based results in order to make a contribution to your field of practice and to the development of the knowledge base of your discipline/practice
Chapter 6: Project analysis and conclusions	Critically review the methodology you used in the project, reflecting on learning achieved and continuing. The presentation of an overview of the project with clear conclusion.
References	These must conform to your university' referencing presentation style; be accurate and complete in both the text and the reference list.
Appendices	These should only provide additional evidence; the main body of work should be complete without them (these do not contribute to the word count).

10 Critically reflect on your project activity and learning and its contribution to your future practice/role.

The structure of postgraduate evidence-based practice dissertations can vary and you should follow any guidelines you are given. However, Table 2.2 provides a typical outline.

Conclusion

Just like you, Sue and Sam are facing the next challenge in their academic journey – the completion of the dissertation. There is something about the dissertation that unsettles the two friends, which might be related to the size of the assignment or the freedom in choosing a project title. In reality, the dissertation gives great freedom in choosing what excites you, the practitioner reader. The remainder of this book explores some essential principles that each will have to follow in developing their ideas and completing the evidence-based practice dissertation.

For further resources for this chapter visit the companion website at
   www.wiley.com/go/glasper/nursingdissertation

Chapter 3 Clinical effectiveness and evidence-based practice: background and history

Alan Glasper[1] and Colin Rees[2]
[1]*University of Southampton, UK*
[2]*University of Cardiff, UK*

Scenario

Sue has attended the first class of her dissertation module that provides the background to evidence-based practice (EBP). She and Sam have got together with their laptops to trace for themselves the origins of evidence-based practice. The clinical environments in which they (and you!) work now expect all staff to understand not only how to access up-to-date publications pertinent to changes in clinical practice, but also to understand the process through which new evidence is generated. Sue and Sam are trying to discover why the system is so important and how it all began.

Introduction

Although evidence-based practice (EBP) seems to have been part of the healthcare nomenclature for some time, it is in fact a relatively new guiding principle within healthcare. As it will underpin so much of what we cover in this book, we start this chapter with a brief background to EBP and its development. It was Sackett *et al.* (1997) who were among the early protagonists of what is now referred to as the evidence-based practice movement (Bick and Graham, 2010). Their definition '*the conscientious, explicit and judicious use of current best evidence about the care of individual patients*' (Sackett *et al.*, 1997:2) has become the accepted mantra of the healthcare professions.

As the patient advocate, nurses owe it to their patients to strive for care based on best evidence. Indeed, the professional regulators for the healthcare professions, such as the Nursing and Midwifery Council (NMC), have at

---

How to Write Your Nursing Dissertation, First Edition. Alan Glasper and Colin Rees.
© 2013 John Wiley & Sons, Ltd. Published 2013 by John Wiley & Sons, Ltd.

the heart of their constitution the protection of the public. The connection between these two ideals of protecting the public and the process of evidence-based practice has been outlined by Fineout-Overholt et al. (2005). Their work details the way nurses and other healthcare professionals can embrace the steps of EBP using a problem solving approach to clinical care that embodies Sackett's principles. The combination of up-to-date best evidence from well-planned studies, health professional know-how and patient preferences and wishes can facilitate optimum evidence-based care.

Historical aspects of evidence-based practice

Ancient civilisations undoubtedly attempted to base their medical practice on the best evidence available at the time. Interestingly, Reid (2008) suggests that the first controlled trail is cited in the bible in the Book of Daniel. Here, Chapter 1, verses 1 through to 21 clearly describe the comparison between two groups of children: one group eating the royal food, namely meat and wine of the King Nebuchadnezzar, and the second comparison group of children who received a vegetarian diet in the form of pulses and who drank only water. The aim of this comparative trial was to establish differences in 'countenance', which usually refers to appearance, especially of the face, and how it is perceived by others.

During this first biblical trial an unknown number of non-royal Israeli children and some of royal birth who were blemish free, wise, able to learn a language and with an understanding of science were given the food and drink of the conquering Persian King whose aim, presumably, was to eradicatedissent against the invaders by making some of these children part of his own royal court. Importantly, the gender mix of these groups was not stated.

The story unfolds that the boy Daniel and three other royal Israeli children, presumably to avoid breaking kosher laws, requested permission from the king's officer, the prince of the eunuchs, 'not to defile himself' with the 'daily rations from the king's food and from the wine he drank' (Kaptchuk and Kerr, 2004). According to the bible, the prince of the eunuchs was very fond of Daniel, who was able to persuade him to undertake what was in effect a 10-day prospective comparative study. Daniel's group of four boys ate pulses (beans) and drank water and the remainder ate the king's food. After the 10 days, Daniel and the three other Israeli royal boys of royal blood had a better countenance than the other Israeli children who enjoyed the diet of the king.

Although this first trial is frequently referred to within the annals of evidence-based practice, Stolberg et al. (2004) have some concerns about it, not least being the lack of science in the randomisation of the individuals participating in the trial. This is important as, without it, there could have been biasing factors (that is, characteristics that might distort the results) in the physical make-up of the two groups and this might have influenced the outcome rather than the type of food. The other major problem you might have considered is the lack of a measure of 'countenance' and how comparisons could have objectively been made between the two groups.

History has also provided other examples of attempts to produce 'evidence' to answer clinical questions. Harvie (2002) describes how Lind, a young naval surgeon's assistant, conducted the first controlled clinical trial in the quest to discover the cause of scurvy, a condition caused by nutritional deficiency that killed many sailors and passengers on long voyages in the 1700s. In 1747, Lind conducted a trial on 12 men with scurvy where one group (n=2) received two oranges and one lemon a day. These two men made a good recovery, whereas the others who were given non-citrus treatments, including sea water, consequently did not recover. Despite the evidence, it was to be another 48 years before the British admiralty began to issue lemon juice to naval seamen for the prevention of scurvy.

Box 3.1 Why the English are called Limeys?

It would have been logical to have nicknamed the English Lemonies after their conquest of scurvy. However, by the mid-nineteenth century the British government decided to spend its resources on West Indian limes rather than Mediterranean lemons, believing that limes were very similar to lemons. Tragically, the amount of vitamin C in limes is significantly less than in lemons, and scurvy returned to blight the British Royal Navy. Although the North Americans still refer to the British as Limeys, had a true randomised controlled trial been conducted, they would in all probability now be called 'Rosies'. WHY?

The answer is that rose hips contain vast amounts of vitamin C and are freely available in the British countryside!

The contribution of the nursing profession to evidence-based practice

Within nursing, the use of data as a source of decision making can be traced back to Florence Nightingale (McDonald, 2001) who powerfully demonstrated her commitment to systematic data collection. After her return from the Crimean war, Nightingale was haunted by the excessive loss of life, mainly caused by disease and not bullets by a factor of seven. She began to lobby for a real investigation into the root cause of this and began to analyse and present data in a way that even a non-statistician could understand. Her work was illustrated with the use of diagrams and Nightingale is credited with the development of colour-coded bar charts and pie charts to illustrate her findings on the death rates of soldiers from infection. Her ability to be ahead of her time is also illustrated by her use of this approach to data collection and presentation to highlight the benefits of a trained nursing workforce compared to that of an untrained workforce (McDonald, 2001).

The 1944 Patulin (a derivative of penicillin) trial for the treatment of the common cold and the 1948 streptomycin trial for tuberculosis were both designed with true randomisation and controls in place (Kaptchuk and Kerr, 2004).The era of modern evidence-based practice was about to begin.

How is evidence sourced?

Evidence-based practice (EBP) is a thoughtful integration of the best available evidence coupled with clinical expertise and the patient's wishes. As such, it enables health practitioners of all varieties to address healthcare questions with an evaluative and quantitative approach. EBP allows the practitioner to assess current and past research, clinical guidelines and other information resources to identify relevant literature, while differentiating between high quality and low quality findings. The practice of evidence-based practice includes six fundamental steps. Melnyk *et al.* (2010) indicate that these include the following:

Step 1: Formulate a Question: this can be achieved using the PICO or similar format (outlined in a later chapter).

Step 2: Find the Evidence: by interrogating research databases such as MEDLINE, CINAHL, Cochrane, Joanna Briggs and so on, not forgetting grey literature (Chapters 6 and 7).

Step 3: Appraise the Evidence: using one of the many critiquing tools available to undertake critical appraisal. This book will concentrate on only three tools (Parahoo, CASP and Rees). However, Melnyk *et al.* (2010) advise nurses who are busy to initially use what they calls Rapid Critical Appraisal, which uses three key questions to allow a quick evaluation of what a particular paper offers:

- *Are the results of the study valid?*
- *What are the results and are they important?*
- *Will the results help me care for my patients?*

Step 4: Integrate the Evidence: this should be combined with clinical expertise and patient preferences and values in applying the evidence. After the studies have been critiqued the next step is to determine the value of the evidence by synthesising their combined weight to check if they all come to a similar conclusion that will warrant a change in clinical practice. Unfortunately, making changes in practice is not a simple process; a full appraisal of how evidence-based health care is implemented in practice is discussed in Chapter 20.

Step 5: Evaluate the Results: here it is crucially important to audit any changes in patient outcomes or service delivery as a result of changes made. This is to ensure that any perceived encouraging effects can be sustained and any harmful effects addressed and prevented.

Step 6: Disseminate the Results: nurses are able to make substantial changes to patient care as a result of their evidence-based practice but sometimes they forget to share their knowledge with others. Part of the whole process is to disseminate knowledge to help other benefit from it. In Chapter 21 details are given on how to use practical methods for disseminating evidence to others from report writing to delivering a paper at a conference.

Conclusion

Evidence-based nursing is the hallmark of professional care and the quest by successive governments to deliver the highest quality care at the optimum cost is likely to drive the profession towards seeking an improved evidence base to underpin and justify its practice. To help, the Chief Nurse for England (NHS, 2010) has produced a series of eight case studies highlighting how nurses can improve quality by making changes to care based on best evidence. Glasper (2010) has indicated that the old adage 'that in god we trust, all other must bring data' applies just as much to the profession of nursing as it does to medicine. Measurement is a central principle of evidence-based practice and accurate measurement enhances decision making in all aspects of heathcare.

References

Bick, D. and Graham, I. (2010) *Evaluating the Impact of Implementing Evidence-Based Practice*. John Wiley & Sons Ltd, Chichester.

Fineout-Overholt, E., Melnyk, B.M. and Schultz, A (2005) Transforming Health Care from the Inside Out: Advancing Evidence-Based Practice in the 21st Century. *Journal of Professional Nursing*, **21** (6), 335–344.

Glasper, E.A. (2010) Can high-impact nursing actions result in enhanced patient care? *British Journal of Nursing*, **19** (6), 1056–1057.

Harvie, D. (2002) Limeys. *The true story of one man's war against Ignorance, the Establishment and the deadly Scurvy*. Sutton Publishing, Stroud, UK.

Kaptchuk, T.J. and Kerr, R.E. (2004) Commentary: Unbiased divination, unbiased evidence, and the Patulin clinical trial. *International Journal of Epidemiology*, **33** (2), 247–251.

McDonald, L. (2001) Florence Nightingale and the early origins of evidence-based nursing. *Evidence Based Nursing Notebook*, **4**, 68–69.

Melnyk, B.M., Fineout-Overholt, E., Stillwell, S. and Williamson, K.M. (2010) Evidence-Based Practice: Step by Step: The Seven Steps of Evidence-Based Practice. *American Journal of Nursing*, **110** (1), 51–53.

NHS (2010) High Impact Actions for Nursing and Midwifery: The Essential Collection. NHS Institute for Innovation and Improvement, Coventry.

Reid, S. (2008) Nothing new under the sun. *Evidence-Based Mental Health*, **11** (2), 33–34.

Sackett, D.L., Rosenberg, W.M.C. and Haynes, R.B. (1997) *Evidence based medicine. How to teach EBM*. Churchill Livingstone, Edinburgh.

Stolberg, H.O., Norman, G. and Trop, I. (2004) Fundamentals of clinical research for radiologists. Randomised controlled trials. *American Journal of Roentgenology*, **183**, 1539–1544.

For further resources for this chapter visit the companion website at
  www.wiley.com/go/glasper/nursingdissertation

Chapter 4   What is evidence-based practice and clinical effectiveness?

Andrée le May
University of Southampton, UK

Scenario

Sue has been to one of the introductory lectures of the top-up degree programme and she and Sam are beginning to see how evidence is becoming integral to contemporary nursing practice.

This chapter is divided into three inter-linked sections. In the first section we will consider the meaning of clinical effectiveness. In the second part the focus will turn to evidence-based practice, a component of clinical effectiveness. In the third section we will concentrate on how care may be made more effective.

Clinical effectiveness

What is clinical effectiveness?

Clinical effectiveness is about providing the best possible healthcare to people within the resources available. In 1996, the UK Department of Health (DH, 1996) defined clinical effectiveness as:

'The extent to which specific clinical interventions when deployed in the field for a particular patient or population do what they are intended to do, i.e.: maintain and improve health and secure the greatest possible health gain from the available resources'.

That same year, the Royal College of Nursing described clinical effectiveness as building on audit and quality improvement in order to provide a

---

How to Write Your Nursing Dissertation, First Edition. Alan Glasper and Colin Rees.
© 2013 John Wiley & Sons, Ltd. Published 2013 by John Wiley & Sons, Ltd.

'framework for linking research, implementation and evaluation in clinical practice' (RCN, 1996:3). This framework has more recently been portrayed, at a more personal level, by NHS Quality Improvement Scotland (NHS QIS 2005) as 'the right person (you) doing:

- the right thing (evidence-based practice)
- in the right way (skills and competence)
- at the right time (providing treatment/services when the patient needs them)
- in the right place (location of treatment/services)
- with the right result (clinical effectiveness/maximising health gain).'

Le May (2012:136–137) suggests that 'in order to do this we need to:

- *have information available* not only about the care that is being delivered – its effectiveness and efficiency – but also any new research evidence about the best care to provide and the best ways through which care could be delivered;
- *openly scrutinise the delivery of care*: practitioners, managers and support workers always need to be thinking about what they do and how they could do things better or more safely; this process needs to be logical and reviewed by others within the team providing health (and social) care – it is the opposite to practising traditionally or ritualistically – a criticism that is made of some nurses;
- *include people who use health-care services* in this process: service users are key drivers for clinical effectiveness and it is important to try wherever possible to co-design services with them (Bates and Robert, 2006); the Picker Institute Europe published a set of principles related to patient-centred care that should be kept in mind when anyone is thinking about clinical effectiveness – it focuses on:
  - respect for patients' values, preference and expressed needs
  - coordination and integration of care
  - information, communication and education
  - physical comfort
  - emotional support and alleviation of fear and anxiety
  - involvement of family and friends
  - continuity and transition
  - access to care.

Activity 4.1

Access the Picker Institute website (http://pickerinstitute.org/about/picker-principles/) where you will find more information about each of these principles and a series of short video clips.

- *identify where change is needed* and ensure that that change is based on evidence either from research, examples of best practice from elsewhere or audit; change should be managed in a purposeful way to make its implementation as effective and efficient as possible;
- *ensure that all change is evaluated* to determine the extent of its success and altered if need be;
- *tell others about what has been done* either through publications or formal/informal presentations; failure to do this maybe why information about the best care often fails to get across to everyone who needs to know and why care in some areas stagnates.

This process needs to be done by everyone. Clinical effectiveness is not just the concern of those providing direct patient care, it needs to be the concern of their managers and their managers too – in other words … clinical effectiveness needs to be a concern of everyone in every organisation (or group of organisations) that provides health and social care.'

Although thinking about clinical effectiveness and trying to make care more clinically effective are not new ideas. Achieving clinical effectiveness can be hard to do in reality. Difficulties are not only associated with the often complex process of understanding care, evaluating its effectiveness and changing it when needed but also with resistance to change and feelings of discomfort when people believe that the care that they have given is effective when it is not.

Clinical effectiveness, in summary, comprises five key components; these are:

1 Having *a way of thinking* that questions care delivery and makes everyone want to know how effective care has been for each person/group of people receiving it. This way of thinking will have started to develop during your initial nursing education – and, of course, is developing even now as you read this book! But once you have left your studies behind, it still needs to continue to develop and be used to promote environments that encourage quality improvement.

2 Using *evidence usually from research or research-based guidelines* to support practice. This can be a challenge – there is SO much evidence out there to select from, which interventions will be effective? A good place to start would be to check out the evidence that is collected on various databases (e.g. the TRIP database http://www.tripdatabase.com/ or at the Joanna Briggs Institute http://www.joannabriggs.edu.au) and of course any National Institute for Health and Clinical Excellence (NICE) (http://www.nice.org.uk/) or Scottish Intercollegiate Guidelines Network (SIGN) (http://www.sign.ac.uk/) guidelines related specifically to the care you are proposing to give. You need to appraise this evidence and decide if it is

clinically relevant to your practice. (Chapter 6 gives more details on how to search for evidence-based literature.)

3   Having the *knowledge, skills and competence* to deliver that research-based care to patients appropriately (at the right time and in the right place): this includes trying to find out if the patient will stick to the pre-scribed care. From time to time the best research-based care does not work because we forget to tailor it to the patient's wider life and previous experiences. Sometimes, despite clear information and instructions, patients do not stick with the care we prescribe (e.g. leaving a particular dressing in place for a given length of time) because it does not suit them in some way. Understanding this – the 'burden' for them that care can create – is important to ensuring its success. If the effort of sticking to the care prescribed (e.g. living with side effects and restrictions on daily life) outweighs the benefits of that care then the patient and their carers are likely to deviate from the care that is planned.

4   Having *an ability to evaluate practice* both at an individual level through evaluations of the success (or not) of daily care and at a group level through audit. This relies on setting clear outcome measures related to care – what do you, the patient and their carer(s) expect to achieve? These should be, wherever possible, shared objectives between the patient/carer and the multidisciplinary team. Only when you make the outcomes of care clear can care be measured in any meaningful way. Sometimes this measurement will rely on pre-determined highly specific tools (e.g. the Edinburgh post-natal depression scale, the SF-36 health measure or the MEWS medical early warning system), sometimes it will depend on less structured observations of improvement (e.g. level of independence) and sometimes on much more qualitative data, in the form of patient stories for instance.

Activity 4.2

See The Mayo Clinic website (http://www.mayoclinic.org/patientstories/) and source a copy and read Gullick and Shimadry's (2008) paper in the *Nursing Times* (this can usually be accessed through your university Learning Resources Centre's online resources, such as electronic journals and online databases).

In your study group discuss the implications and veracity of these patient stories.

---

5   Having or developing *a commitment to disseminating* how effective care has been, and either formally or informally communicating this to others.

Evidence-based practice

For well over 25 years, prominence has been given to the use of research evidence in healthcare in an attempt to further increase clinical effectiveness and the quality of care delivered to patients. Many definitions have been provided for evidence-based medicine/healthcare/practice but the one that best characterises the push for the use of research evidence in nursing comes from Cullum *et al.* (2008:2), who define evidence-based nursing as 'the application of valid, relevant research-based information in nurse decision making'.

Whilst noting the importance of applying valid and relevant research to practice, it is important to remember that rigorous and relevant research may not always be available to base practice on. If this is the case, practitioners need to consider what other sorts of evidence could be used to support effective and efficient care. Other sources of evidence might include:

- Evidence based on structured evaluations of practice (audit or other analyses of safety records, complaints etc.)
- Evidence based on theory which is not grounded in research.
- Evidence based on our experiences (professional and general).
- Evidence gathered from our clients/patients and/or their carers.
- Evidence passed on to us by role models experts.
- Evidence based on policy directives.

Sometimes none of these is relevant and we have to search more widely for knowledge to help us to provide appropriate care. This might include searching for unpublished evidence in reports, research abstracts or conference proceedings using the internet or finding, as Sue has done in the scenario, information available in the media. Evidence emanating from the media needs particularly careful appraisal before implementation with thorough follow-up of any primary sources referred to. If none is available you can check out any evidence base behind the article by using the website 'Behind the Headlines' (http://www.nhs.uk/news/Pages/NewsIndex.aspx). This web-site gives 'you the facts without the fiction' and can be accessed by healthcare practitioners and patients. If you still need more information contact the reporter.

Practising in an evidence-based practice way is usually described as a fairly simple linear process (Box 4.1). Of course, it is never as simple as it appears in theory and we will discuss this more later in Chapter 5.

Attention needs to be paid to establishing the rigour of the evidence – research or otherwise. For research evidence this is primarily about reliability and validity. There are many guides and tools that can help you do this (e.g. the series of critical appraisal tools available at the Centre for Evidence Based

> **Box 4.1**   The process of evidence-based healthcare (adapted from Sackett *et al.* 2004).
>
> 1. Asking clear questions about practice – usually about an individual patient.
> 2. Looking for answers to those questions – firstly searching for research findings.
> 3. Judging (critically appraising) the evidence for its rigour, validity (truthfulness) and usefulness to practice.
> 4. Integrating these findings with clinical expertise, patient needs, patient preferences.
> 5. If appropriate, applying these findings to the patient's care.
> 6. Evaluating the outcome of our decisions/ practice.

Medicine (CEBM) http://www.cebm.net/?o=1157) and advice is given in Sections 4 and 5 of this book. For other sorts of evidence le May and Gabbay (2011) have constructed a useful set of pointers (Table 4.1).

Once you've decided that the evidence is reliable and valid it is important to establish its clinical relevance. This should be done by asking a set of questions (le May, 1999; le May and Gabbay, 2011). For example:

Is the evidence relevant clinically for the client?

1   What benefits will the implementation of this evidence have for patients/carers/staff?

2   What risks are associated with implementation/non-implementation?

Can the evidence be used by the organisation within which care is being given?

1   Are there enough resources for implementation?

2   What are the opportunities for and constraints to implementing this evidence?

Once you have established that the evidence can be trusted and is clinically relevant to your client then the implementation process can begin (Section 6).

Making care more effective

Clinical effectiveness is embedded in our healthcare system, from the commissioning of services to the delivery of care. Earlier we said that clinical effectiveness had developed from audit and quality improvement – these links still remain, but it is also important to have the right evidence available as well as access to supportive organisational structures – for instance those supporting clinical governance. We will come back to the challenges faced by practitioners who are trying to get research into practice in Chapter 5.

Own experiences	Theoretical perspectives (non-research based)	Client's/Patient's/Carer's experiences	Role model's/expert's opinions	Policy directives
Relevance to the clinical issue	**Link between theory and clinical issue**	**Relevance to the current situation**	**Depth and breadth of expertise**	**Type and strength of evidence used to support directive(s)**
Frequency/uniqueness of experience	Strengths and weaknesses of argument being presented	Frequency/uniqueness of experience	Credibility	Relevance to current situation or clinical issue
Extent to which experiences have been shared by others	What sources of evidence are used?	Extent to which experiences have been shared by others	Reason for choice – what defines expertise?	Currency – date when last reviewed
Extent to which other sources of evidence support experiences	Credibility	Extent to which other sources of evidence support experiences	What sources of evidence are drawn upon to support knowledge?	Likelihood of transferability to practice setting
Extent of transferability of experiences to current situation	Appropriateness of theory to clinical issue	Richness of the description	Relevance of advice to current situation	Evidence of use elsewhere or evaluation of impact
	Appropriateness of recommendations for practice	**Extent of transferability of experiences to current situation**	Likelihood of transferability of evidence to practice setting	
	Likelihood of transferability to practice setting		Evidence of use elsewhere or evaluation of impact	
	Evidence of use elsewhere or evaluation of impact			

There are many mechanisms already used for making care more effective – some are more directive and distant from the front line of care delivery than others. The more directive approaches include:

- Following guidance published by NICE, SIGN or a professional body such as the RCN or RCM. The extent to which care conforms to these guidelines may be measured through external audits in the form of inspections by the Care Quality Commission (http://www.cqc.org.uk/) or internal organisational audits.
- Through contractual incentives, for example Quality Outcomes Framework (QOF) of General Practitioners' contracts. This awards points (and associated funding) to practices for achieving specific outcomes (for further details see http://www.nice.org.uk/aboutnice/qof/qof.jsp).
- Through regulation – the NMC sets standards / competencies against which practitioners deliver care.
- By monitoring care against explicit standards through organisational audits carried out by the Care Quality Commission with the purpose of promoting improvement in health and healthcare.

The less centrally directed ones tend to involve healthcare workers and service users in understanding the process of care – often described as the patient's journey through the healthcare system. These techniques have become increasingly sophisticated, systematised and have been given stranger and stranger names over the last fifteen years! Some examples that you may be familiar with include the Deming Cycle – better known as the **P**lan, **D**o, **S**tudy, **A**ct cycle (PDSA) and Lean thinking. Originally developed from the car making industry they are now being successfully used in healthcare settings across the world to analyse and improve the process of care delivery and its outcome for patients (and staff). Despite using different methods (Box 4.2) they essentially aim to do one thing – help us determine if the care given to patients is as good as it possibly could be and, if not, they provide us with ways to identify how care could be improved.

Making care more effective relies on everyone involved taking responsibility for its delivery, alteration and evaluation. This process needs to blend the systematic study of the process of care – either in one part of the organisation (e.g. the ward, the team or the unit) or across the organisation(s) (e.g. the hospital, the Trust, the health economy) – with evidence-based decision making. Whilst a range of quality improvement techniques are available to steer this process, undertaking it will also rely on some or all of the following:

- the provision of continuing educational opportunities following qualification;
- the use of skilled, inclusive leadership that engages everyone necessary;
- the harnessing of patients' and other lay representatives' views;

Box 4.2 Summaries of the PDSA cycle and LEAN thinking (from le May, 2012:140–141).

The **PDSA cycle**, popularised by the Institute for Healthcare Improvement (IHI) (http://www.ihi.org/IHI/) in North America, has been used across the world in order to make improvements to healthcare. Essentially, it is about finding the answers to three key questions – What are we trying to accomplish? What change can we make that will result in an improvement? How will we know that a change is an improvement? The cycle is used to 'test a change by developing a plan to test the change (Plan), carrying out the test (Do), observing and learning from the consequences (Study), and determining what modifications should be made to the test (Act)'
(http://www.ihi.org/IHI/Topics/Improvement/ImprovementMethods/Tools/ Plan-Do-Study-Act%20(PDSA)%20Worksheet).
The PDSA cycle is most often associated with small scale change at particular hot spots in an organisation or a particular care pathway. Although we often read about PDSA being used by healthcare workers it can be effectively used by volunteers or lay carers. Maurice Wilson (2005) a volunteer with the Healthy Communities Collaborative in Northampton writes about what it was like to use the PDSA cycle to help change services within his local community. The collaborative used the PDSA cycle to place the onus for action on the community volunteers and by doing this enabled them 'to work in equal partnership with health professions. The beauty of the project was that it was 'action-based', which meant success rested with community volunteers themselves: it was about people feeling included in any change and their contributions and opinions being valued' (Wilson, 2005:127).
LEAN thinking is often described as a way of achieving larger scale change across an organisation(s) and takes a somewhat different approach to the PDSA cycle. Refined by Toyota this approach has been adapted for use in healthcare (Miller, 2005; DH, UK Department of Health, 2008) but probably the best known use of LEAN thinking in nursing is the work undertaken on the 'Productive Ward' initiative supported by the Institute for Innovation and Improvement from 2007. LEAN thinking seeks essentially to do more with less (http://www.lean.org/) – the emphasis being to strip out waste from the system so that care can be provided, to the highest possible standard, in the most cost effective way. Various techniques are used within the LEAN thinking process (for a useful summary of these go to
http://www.atoshealthcare.com/UserFiles/File/fact-sheets/2642-0609%20 Achieving%20Lean%20and%20healthy%20transformation%20FS.pdf).
Sometimes LEAN thinking is linked to Six Sigma – a very quantitative approach. Six Sigma has five phases – define, measure, analyse, improve and control (DMAIC). The first phase includes a cost–benefit analysis and only if this is acceptable should the project progress any further. In the measurement phase, baseline data are collected to help the project team understand and quantify what is happening at the outset – this information can then be used to design a solution which will improve care and produce measurable outcomes that will show success at subsequent monitoring (for more information go to http://www.isixsigma.com).

> **Box 4.3**   Tips for thinking about clinical effectiveness in your healthcare
> dissertation.
>
> When writing your dissertation remember:
> • to emphasise how understanding your topic better could help improve
>   clinical effectiveness;
> • that your question may not be answered by finding research-based evidence
>   on its own;
> • to tell your readers what other sources of evidence you used to help you find
>   out about your topic and how you appraised these pieces of evidence.

• the use of guidelines to guide and change practice;
• the use of local opinion leaders and champions;
• the allocation of protected time;
• the use of audit or other quality improvement techniques and feedback;
• the availability and use of profile raising units (e.g. the NHS Institute for
  Innovation and Improvement in England (http://www.institute.nhs.uk/),
  the Institute for Health Improvement in North America (http://www.ihi.
  org/IHI/), The Health Foundation in England (http://www.health.org.uk/));
• creating ways for people to meet in order to talk about practice and how to
  make it more effective.

Tips for thinking about clinical effectiveness in your healthcare dissertation
are shown in Box 4.3.

References

Bates, P. and Robert, G. (2006) Experience-based design: from redesigning the system
around the patient to co-designing services with the patient. *Quality and Safety in
Health Care*, **15**, 307–310.

Behind the Headlines, http://www.nhs.uk/news/Pages/NewsIndex.aspx (last accessed
16th October 2010).

Care Quality Commission, http://www.cqc.org.uk/ (last accessed 16 October 2010).

CASP, http://www.phru.nhs.uk/casp/casp.htm (last accessed 16 October 2010).

Cullum, N., Cilisha, D., Maynes, B. nad Marks, S. (2008) *Evidence-based nursing: an
introduction*. Blackwell Publishing, Oxford.

DH (UK Department of Health) (1996) *Promoting clinical effectiveness a framework
for action in and through the NHS*. The Stationery Office, London.

DH (UK Department of Health) (2008) *High Quality Care for All: NHS Next Stage
Review Final Report*. The Stationery Office, London.

Gullick, J. and Shimadry, B. (2008) Using patient stories to improve quality of care.
Nursing Times, **104**, 10, 33–34.

Institute for Health Improvement, http://www.ihi.org/IHI/ (last accessed 16 October
2010).

Joanna Briggs Institute, http://www.joannabriggs.edu.au (last accessed 16 October 2010).

le May, A. (1999) *Evidence Based Practice*. Nursing Times Clinical Monograph No 1. EMAP, London.

le May, A. (2012) Evaluating Care. (Chapter 11) In: A. le May and S. Holmes *Introduction to Nursing Research: Developing Research Awareness*. Hodder Arnold, London.

le May, A. and Gabbay, J. (2011) Evidence-based practice: more than research needed? In: G. Lewith, J. Cousins, and H. Walach (eds), *Clinical research in complementary therapies*. Churchill Livingstone: Elsevier, Edinburgh.

Mayo Clinic, http://www.mayoclinic.org/patientstories/ (last accessed 16 October 2010).

Miller, D. (2005) *Going Lean in Health Care*. Institute for Healthcare Improvement, Cambridge, MA.

National Institute for Health and Clinical Excellence, http://www.nice.org.uk/ (last accessed 16 October 2010).

NHS Institute for Innovation and Improvement, http://www.institute.nhs.uk/ (last accessed 16 October 2010).

NHS QIS (2005), http://www.clinicalgovernance.scot.nhs.uk/section2/definition.asp (last accessed 16 October 2010).

Picker Institute Europe, http://pickerinstitute.org/about/picker-principles/ (last accessed 16th October 2010).

RCN (1996) *Clinical Effectiveness*. Royal College of Nursing, London.

Sackett, D., Strauss, S., Richardson, W., Rosenberg, W. and Haynes, R. (2004) *Evidence based medicine: how to practice and teach EBM*. Churchill Livingstone, London.

Scottish Intercollegiate Guidelines Network, http://www.sign.ac.uk/ (last accessed 16 October 2010).

The Health Foundation, http://www.health.org.uk/ (last accessed 16 October 2010).

TRIP database, http://www.tripdatabase.com/ (last accessed 16 October 2010).

Wilson, M. (2005) Preventing falls in older people. In: M. Rawlins and P. Littlejohns (eds), *Delivering Quality in the NHS*. Radcliffe, Oxford.

For further resources for this chapter visit the companion website at
www.wiley.com/go/glasper/nursingdissertation

Chapter 5 The challenges of delivering practice based on best evidence (in primary, secondary and tertiary settings)

Andrée le May
University of Southampton, UK

Scenario

Sue has already had meaningful ideas about evidence-based practice and she and Sam have been considering just what constitutes best evidence.

Chapter 4 of this book emphasised the importance of clinical effectiveness and evidence-based practice. This chapter considers the challenges of delivering practice based on the best available evidence. The chapter is divided into three sections: the first section reminds readers that practice is underpinned by many sorts of evidence; the second section details the barriers that may well stop practitioners, regardless of their clinical speciality, from using research evidence in their practice; and the final section identifies ways through which the use of research-based practice can be encouraged and suggests ways to overcome some of the known barriers to research implementation.

An evidence base for practice

Every nurse needs to make every effort to use, as Cullum *et al.* (2008:2) put it, 'valid, relevant research-based information in (their) decision making', since delivering research-based care is central to achieving clinical effectiveness. However, doing this is not as simple as it may at first appear. This may sometimes be because there simply is no research-based information available

---

How to Write Your Nursing Dissertation, First Edition. Alan Glasper and Colin Rees.
© 2013 John Wiley & Sons, Ltd. Published 2013 by John Wiley & Sons, Ltd.

and other sorts of information have to be used, or the research evidence exists but cannot be found or if it can be found it cannot be used because it does not fit with patients' preferences or because the healthcare organisation does not have the necessary resources to implement it. Any or all of these factors may be further complicated by a process whereby research-based information is melded with other sorts of information, rendering its original state unidentifiable (Gabbay *et al.*, 2003; le May, 2009). This transformation makes it not only hard for practitioners to identity and articulate specific research findings that have informed their practice but also for others interested in the implementation of research to work out how much research is actually being used.

We can be sure, though, from research and from listening to nurses, that in the complex reality of practice nurses do not only use research-based information to guide their practice; they use many sorts of evidence in order to provide high quality care (le May, 1999). More specifically, Rycroft-Malone *et al.* (2004) outlined four types of evidence that underpinned the delivery of care – research, clinical experience, patient experience and information from the local context. A year later Estabrooks *et al.* (2005) expanded this list demonstrating, through two case studies, that nurses' practical knowledge was obtained from their social interactions with others, their experiences, documents and a priori knowledge. Additionally, Estabrooks *et al.* (2005:460) suggested that these findings challenged the 'disproportionate weight that proponents of the evidence-based movement ascribe to research knowledge'. More recently Mills *et al.* (2009) found in a survey of 590 Australian general practice nurses that they found experiential learning and interactions with clients, peers, medical practitioners and specialist nurses of greater importance to their practice than knowledge found in research journals.

In opposition to this view Profetto-McGrath *et al.* (2007) found that whilst Canadian clinical nurse specialists accessed and used evidence from many sources they indicated that research literature was a primary source of evidence and research was used in their decision making, with the choice of evidence often depending on the type of question they were answering. In addition to evidence gathered from 'front line' nurses, healthcare team members and families the clinical nurse specialists used the Internet to search research databases and other online sources of evidence as well as using it to communicate with peers and ask questions about current practice. Gerrish *et al.'s* (2008) survey of nurses in two hospitals in England found that they, too, relied heavily on personal experience and communication with colleagues rather than formal sources of knowledge. However, they also found differences in levels of seniority with the more senior nurses being more confident generally in accessing research and changing practice. This may well support Profetto-McGrath *et al*.'s (2007) positive findings about clinical nurse specialists – the two studies together suggesting that the more senior the practitioner the more able they are in seeking out research-based information and implementing change based on it. All of these findings reflect the realities of practice experienced by many nurses today.

The findings from Gabbay and le May's (2004, 2011) ethnographic observations of GPs, practice nurses and medical students throw further light on the conundrum of research use in practice showing that, and explaining how, practitioners bring together many types of knowledge in order to form a very broad evidence base for high quality care; they called this amalgam 'clinical mindlines'. Clinical mindlines are:

'… *internalised, collectively reinforced and often tacit guidelines that are informed by clinicians' training, by their own and each others' experience, by their interactions with their role sets, by their reading, by the way they have learnt to handle the(ir) conflicting demands, by their understanding of local circumstances and systems, and by a host of other sources … Clinicians build up mindlines as a bank of personalised, flexible syntheses of all the different types of theoretical and experiential knowledge that they need to be able to call upon instantaneously.*'

(Gabbay and le May, 2011:43–44).

Gabbay and le May (2004) also found that practitioners only briefly 'grazed' the research literature, paying minimal attention to this source of evidence as a way of informing their practice. This does not mean that practice was poor – on the contrary, care was excellent in the practices observed – neither does it mean that decisions were not based on research-based information, rather it may simply mean that research journals are not the main ways through which practitioners find out about research.

Barriers to the use of research evidence in practice

Over the last five years more emphasis has been placed by the UK government, the Higher Education Funding Council, the Department of Health and research funders on the need to increase the impact of research 'at the bedside' in order to improve patient care and justify their considerable financial investment in research. Despite a concomitant effort to make research more readily available in guidelines and policy statements, many practitioners would agree, if asked, that nursing decisions are still not always informed by the best and most up-to-date research. But why is this so? Numerous researchers have tried to answer

Box 5.1   Practitioners' perceived barriers to research-based practice (adapted from le May *et al.*, 1998).

Attitudes
• Lack of cooperation
• Lack of motivation
• Fear
• Resistance to change/ritualised practice

Beliefs
• Research will not make a difference
• Research data are not appropriate
• Conviction that current practice is OK

Professional relationship
• Medical staff block implementation
• Medical staff consider nursing research substandard
• Nursing colleagues are uncooperative
• Senior staff are resistant to change
• Research should be undertaken by practitioners
• Research 'goes' with an individual
• Low grading of research staff

Organisational issues
• Time
• Pressure of workload
• Too much change

Educational issues
• Practitioners unaware of or unable to access research
• Lack of skills in critical appraisal
• Research reports are jargonistic

this question, hoping that by identifying barriers to research use they will be able to construct suitable interventions to promote better use of research. Let us take a look at what these barriers are.

Kajermo *et al.* (2010) brought together data from sixty-three research studies that have used the BARRIERS scale to assess barriers to nurses' research use over the last twenty years. This systematic review concludes that the main barriers are related to the setting within which implementation occurs and the presentation of research findings. The authors state that barriers were consistent over time and also location. More extensive qualitative data from a study of practitioners' and managers' cultures of research (le May *et al.*, 1998) suggested that, whilst some barriers do revolve around the setting in which nurses work and the jargon used in the presentation of research findings (Box 5.1), there are other important factors, such as attitudes, beliefs and professional relationships, that need to be considered.

Furthermore, Gerrish *et al*.'s (2008) survey showed distinct differences between junior and senior nurses. Whilst all 598 respondents said they were confident finding and using evidence in practice, the senior nurses not only felt more confident accessing various sources of evidence (e.g. published sources and using the internet) but they also were confident initiating change. Conversely, junior nurses were less confident finding out about their organisation and were less confident implementing change. Lack of time and resources were also noted as major barriers by the more junior nurses but not their senior colleagues, who felt able to overcome these limitations. Barriers cited by clinical nurse specialists in Canada (Profetto-McGrath *et al*., 2007) support previous research and included lack of time, lack of resources and lack of receptivity at both clinical and organisational levels.

There seems then to be some consistency emerging in relation to the barriers identified, with nurses' use of research-based information being affected by several tangible challenges associated with:

- Their work setting – lack of receptivity at clinical and organisational levels
- The way research findings are presented
- Lack of time
- Lack of/inappropriateness of resources.

These may also be influenced by their attitudes and beliefs about research and their own ability to implement change (le May, 2012).

In addition to the barriers detailed above, practitioners sometimes suggest that the wrong research is being done, as the results will not answer the questions that practitioners need answers to. Increasingly, efforts are being made to minimise this mismatch by strengthening interactions between practitioners and researchers in order to fine tune research questions and designs to meet the needs of practice (le May, 2012).

One popular approach to doing this is to use action research which, as Sam explained to Sue over coffee, is about 'engaging staff in research about their own practice enable(ing) them to take ownership of the change'. Sam isn't the only one to think like this – Munten et al.'s (2010) review is testament to the increasing interest being paid to action research as a 'promising' mechanism for implementing evidence-based practice. Another approach is to develop Van de Ven and Johnson's (2006) idea of engaged scholarship, which closely links research to the needs of practice and policy through co-construction (Gabbay and le May, 2011; McCormack, 2011) – this is rather like the idea of action research that excited Sam.

Encouraging the use of research evidence in practice

Knowing the barriers that nurses face in using research should make it easier to design interventions to help them. A quick search through the literature (le May, 2012) reveals that over the last twenty years many different approaches have been used to encourage nurses around the world to use research evidence in practice, with varying degrees of success. Given this huge literature a sensible way forward was to find a systematic review in order to provide conclusive evidence of which approaches were best.

Thompson *et al*'s (2007) systematic review is the only one to focus on interventions aimed at increasing research use in nursing. They took a highly structured approach including only the most robust studies available. Although 8000 titles were screened only four studies met the criteria for inclusion – three randomised controlled trials and one controlled 'before and after' study. The principal intervention in all of the four studies was education but it was not just simply providing education that mattered, it was the way that the education was delivered that impacted on its success (or not). When education occurred in researcher-led educational meetings it was ineffective (two studies). However, when a local opinion leader led the educational meeting it was effective (one study) and when the education occurred in multidisciplinary committee meetings around a particular topic (oncology pain) it was also effective (one study). Unfortunately, the restrictive methodology of this systematic review only allows us to say that in some cases education works – in other cases it does not: what it does suggest is that education associated with an environment within which trusted colleagues are present (either as opinion leaders or multidisciplinary team co-workers) may make it more successful.

Education also was an important feature for Profetto-McGrath *et al*'s (2007) sample of clinical nurse specialists in Canada along with peers and organisational support. Organisational support, interprofessional relationships and education also featured in le May *et al*'s (1998) study of nurses and their managers in England – however, so did other interesting factors, namely reorganisations in the NHS and the creation of new structures/fora (Box 5.2).

In relation to these last two points, several reorganisations of the NHS have occurred since this study was completed, with the emergence of new structures that have offered many opportunities for the development of closer links between researchers and practitioners (le May, 2012). Probably the most ambitious of these is the Collaborations for Leadership in Applied Health Research and Care (CLAHRC) initiative developed in 2008 by the National Institute for Health Research (NIHR) at the Department of

---

Box 5.2   Opportunities to develop research-based practice (adapted from le
May *et al.*, 1998).

Organisational support
- Specific research and development strategy for trust or for nursing
- Enhanced links with education providers
- Funding for courses and workshops; award schemes
- Specific appointments
- Identification and support of champions for nursing

New 'structures'
- Research fora
- Research awareness groups
- Proactive research/ethics committees
- Research centre
- Nursing development units

Interprofessional relationships
- Multiprofessional initiatives, e.g. guideline development
- Multidisciplinary research

Changing individuals
- Greater uptake of continuing education
- Recognition of importance of research by individuals
- Project 2000 and degree courses increasing individual skills and knowledge

Reorganised NHS
- Evidence-based purchasing

Health in response to the Cooksey Report (Cooksey, 2006). The CLAHRCs'
primary functions are to conduct high quality applied health research, implement findings from research in clinical practice and increase the capacity of
NHS organisations to engage with and apply research including continuing
professional development (http://clahrc-sy.nihr.ac.uk/about.html).

Alongside this, le May (2012) reminds us that there has been the almost
parallel development of structures within the NHS and the Higher Education
Sector that gave rise to creation of formal Clinical Academic Career pathways
(UKCRC, 2007). Another initiative spearheaded by the NIHR to promote
closer links between research and practice, this encourages practitioners to
stay in practice and develop their research skills by splitting their workload
between delivering care and researching it. This initiative supports the
already established nursing and midwifery consultant posts which have the
remit, although not as explicitly detailed, to link closely the implementation
of research with providing care.

Some researchers, practitioners and academics have put forward models
or frameworks which, if followed, might improve the use of research-based

Box 5.3   The main elements of the most recent Promoting Action on Research Implementation in Health Services (PARiHS) framework (Rycroft-Malone, 2010).

- This framework emphasises that the success of implementation depends on the relationship between key factors:
  1. the nature of the evidence (whether it is research, clinical experience or patient experience);
  2. the context within which it is implemented (this includes the culture of the organisation, leadership and the potential for evaluation);
  3. the ways through which this implementation is facilitated (this depends on the role of the facilitator and their attributes and skills).
- The most successful implementation will occur 'when evidence is scientifically robust and matches professional consensus and patients' preferences … the context receptive to change with sympathetic cultures, strong leadership, and appropriate monitoring and feedback systems … and, when there is appropriate facilitation of change with input from skilled external and internal facilitators' (pages 112–113).
- This framework may be used to diagnose the receptiveness of each context to change and, thereby, tailor any facilitation to meet the needs of that specific context.

Box 5.4   The main elements of the Ottawa Model of Research Use (OMRU) (Logan and Graham, 2010).

- This model specifically focuses on getting valid research findings implemented.
- There are six key structural elements
  1. the research-informed innovation
  2. the potential adopters
  3. the practice environment
  4. implementation interventions for transferring the research findings into practice
  5. the adoption of the innovation
  6. the outcomes – health related and others.
- In addition, there are three process elements (AME) that need to be considered – Assessment of barriers and supports (these are associated with the structural elements 1–3 above), Monitoring how the research-informed innovation is implemented and Evaluation of the impact of the innovation (monitoring and evaluation are linked closely to structural elements 4–6).
- This model can be applied to evidence-based practice projects and also quality improvement projects.

Box 5.5   The main elements of the Knowledge-to-Action (KTA) framework
(Graham and Tetroe, 2010).

This framework is conceptually robust, being derived from an analysis of 31
planned action/change theories in health and social sciences, education and
management.
- The framework emphasises the importance of social interaction and of tailor-
ing evidence to meet contextual and cultural needs.
- The framework comprises a number of phases:
  1. Identify problem/select knowledge
  2. Adapt knowledge to the local context
  3. Assess barriers to knowledge use
  4. Implement tailored intervention
  5. Monitor knowledge use
  6. Evaluate outcomes (both those associated with the process of change and
     the outcomes in relation to healthcare)
  7. Sustain knowledge use.

Box 5.6   The main elements of the Joanna Briggs Institute (JBI) framework
for implementing evidence (Pearson, 2010).

This framework is particularly focused on the use of research evidence.
- At its core there are four key components:
  1. healthcare evidence generation
  2. evidence synthesis
  3. evidence/knowledge transfer
  4. use of evidence.
- Our primary concern is the use of evidence – this part of the framework
  focuses on practice change, embedding evidence through system/organisa-
  tion-wide change and evaluating its impact.
- The framework emphasises that the process of use of evidence is influenced by:
  1. resources
  2. education/expertise
  3. patient preference
  4. the availability of research
  5. staffing levels, skill mix
  6. policies.

---

information in practice. Probably the best known of these are the models
developed and refined over the last 10 years by a team of researchers at the
Royal College of Nursing in the UK – the Promoting Action on Research
Implementation in Health Services (PARiHS) framework (Kitson *et al.*,
1998) – two Canadian teams working to produce the Ottawa Model of Research
Use (OMRU) (Logan and Graham, 2010) and the Knowledge-to-Action (KTA)

model (Graham and Tetroe, 2010) and the Australian Joanna Briggs Institute (JBI) (Pearson, 2010). The main elements of these models are presented in Boxes 5.3–5.6 but further details of these and several other models and frameworks for implementing evidence-based practice are presented in a comprehensive textbook edited by Rycroft-Malone and Bucknall (2010).

In addition to these frameworks, Baker et al.'s (2010) systematic review of 26 studies of interventions that could successfully overcome barriers to change shows us how difficult it is to identify, with any degree of certainty, interventions that really do work. Whilst they indicated that tailored interventions could change professional practice they could not tell us which ones would be the most effective approaches to reducing barriers to change.

Conclusion

Whilst acknowledging that nurses and other healthcare professionals use many types of evidence to underpin effective practice, this chapter has emphasised the importance of research evidence. Implementing research-based information is not as easy as it first appears and the smooth flow of research into practice is often prevented by a series of individual and organisational barriers. However, there is an emerging body of knowledge which suggests that carefully targeted educational interventions, particularly those involving trusted colleagues and/or opinion leaders, may help to overcome some of these barriers. In addition, using participative research designs (e.g. action research) or engaged scholarship, which forges partnerships between researchers and practitioners, can also facilitate a closer match between the research needs of practitioners and the research generated for implementation. The whole process of research use may be structured by one of the many frameworks available. Using one of these frameworks may be helpful when you either come to change practice in your workplace or plan how you might undertake a change to practice, based on the answer to your question, in your dissertation.

References

Baker, R., Camosso-Stefinovic, J., Gillies, C. et al. (2010.) *Tailored interventions to overcome identified barriers to change: effects on professional practice and health care outcomes (Review).*Cochrane Database of Systematic Reviews 2010, Issue 3. Art. No.: CD005470. DOI: 10.1002/14651858.CD005470.pub2.

Cooksey, D. (2006) *A review of UK health funding.* HMSO, Norwich.

Cullum, N., Cilisha, D., Maynes, B. and Marks, S. (2008) *Evidence-based nursing: an introduction.* Blackwell Publishing, Oxford.

Estabrooks, C., Rutakumwa, W., O'Leary, K. *et al.* (2005) Sources of Practice Knowledge among Nurses. *Qualitative Health Research*, **15** (4), 460–476.

Gabbay, J. and le May, A. (2004) Evidence-based guidelines or collectively constructed "mind-lines"? An ethnographic study of knowledge management in primary care. *British Medical Journal*, **329**, 1013–1020.

Gabbay, J. and le May, A. (2011) *Practice Based Evidence for Healthcare: Clinical Mindlines*. Routledge, London.

Gabbay, J., le May, A., Jefferson, H.*et al.* (2003) A case study of knowledge management in multi-agency consumer-informed 'communities of practice': implications for evidence-based policy development in health and social services. *Health*, **7** (3), 283–310.

Gerrish, K., Ashworth, P., Lacey, A. and Bailey, J. (2008) Developing evidence-based practice: experiences of senior and junior clinical nurses. *Journal of Advanced Nursing*, **62** (1), 62–73.

Graham, I. and Tetroe, J. (2010) The Knowledge to Action framework. In: Rycroft-Malone J and Bucknall T (eds), *Models and Frameworks for Implementing Evidence-Based Practice: Linking Evidence to Action*. John Wiley & Sons Ltd, Chichester.

Kajermo, K., Boström, A-M., Thompson, D., Hutchinson, A., Estabrooks, C. and Wallin, L. (2010) The BARRIERS scale – the barriers to research utilization scale: A systematic review. *Implementation Science*, **5**, 32.

Kitson, A.L., Harvey, G. and McCormack, B. (1998) Enabling the implementation of evidence based practice: a conceptual framework. *Quality in Health Care*, **7**, 149–158.

le May, A. (1999) *Evidence Based Practice*. Nursing Times Clinical Monograph No. 1, EMAP, London.

le May, A. (2009) Generating Patient Capital: the contribution of story telling in Communities of Practice designed to develop older people's services. In: A. le May, *Communities of Practice in Health and Social Care*. Blackwell Publishing, Oxford.

le May, A. (2012) Evaluating Care. In: A. le May, A and S. Holmes (eds), *Introduction to Nursing Research: Developing Research Awareness*, Chapter 10. Hodder Arnold, London.

le May, A., Mulhall, A. and Alexander, C. (1998) Bridging the research–practice gap: exploring the research cultures of practitioners and managers. *Journal of Advanced Nursing*, **28** (2), 428–437.

Logan, J. and Graham, I. (2010) The Ottawa Model of Research Use. In: J. Rycroft-Malone and T. Bucknall (eds), *Models and Frameworks for Implementing Evidence-Based Practice: Linking Evidence to Action*. John Wiley & Sons Ltd, Chichester.

McCormack, B. (2011 in press) Engaged Scholarship and research impact: Integrating the doing and using of research in practice. *Journal of Research in Nursing*, **16** (2), 111–127.

Mills, J., Field, J. and Cant, R. (2009) The Place of Knowledge and Evidence in the Context of Australian General Practice Nursing. *Worldviews on Evidence-Based Nursing*, **6**, 219–228.

Munten, G., Van Den Bogaard, J., Cox, K., Garretsen, H. and Bongers, I. (2010) Implementation of Evidence-Based Practice in Nursing Using Action Research:

A Review. *Worldviews on Evidence-Based Nursing*, 7, 135–157. Pearson, A. (2010) The Joanna Briggs Institute model of evidence-based health care as a framework for implementing evidence. In: J. Rycroft-Malone and T. Bucknall (eds), *Models and Frameworks for Implementing Evidence-Based Practice: Linking Evidence to Action*. John Wiley & Sons Ltd, Chichester.

Profetto-McGrath, J., Smith, K., Hugo, K., Taylor, M. and El-Hajj, H. (2007) Clinical Nurse Specialists' Use of Evidence in Practice: A Pilot Study. *Worldviews on Evidence-Based Nursing*, 4, 86–96.

Rycroft Malone, J. (2010) Promoting Action on Research Implementationin Health Services (PARIHS). In: J. Rycroft-Malone and T. Bucknall (eds), *Models and Frameworks for Implementing Evidence-Based Practice: Linking Evidence to Action*. John Wiley & Sons Ltd, Chichester.

Rycroft-Malone, J. and Bucknall, T. (eds) (2010) *Models and Frameworks for Implementing Evidence-Based Practice: Linking Evidence to Action*. John Wiley & Sons Ltd, Chichester.

Rycroft-Malone, J., Seers, K., Titchen, A., Harvey, G., Kitson, A. and McCormack, B. (2004) What counts as evidence in evidence-based practice? *Journal of Advanced Nursing*, **47** (1), 81–90.

Thompson, D., Estabrooks, C., Scott-Findlay, S., Moore, K. and Wallin, L. (2007) Interventions aimed at increasing research use in nursing: a systematic review *Implementation Science*, **2**, 15.

UKCRC (2007) *Developing the best research professionals. Qualified graduate nurses: recommendations for preparing and supporting clinical academic nurses of the future*. Report of the UKCRC Subcommittee for Nurses in Clinical Research (Workforce), United Kingdom Clinical Research Collaboration (UKCRC), London.

Van de Ven, A. and Johnson, P. (2006) Knowledge for theory and practice. *Academy of Management Review*, **31**, 802–821.

For further resources for this chapter visit the companion website at

www.wiley.com/go/glasper/nursingdissertation

Section 2 **Sourcing and accessing evidence for your dissertation**

Sue asks Sam for advice. She has some ideal 'evidence' for her dissertation but it is from a 'Sunday Supplement Magazine'; does this count as evidence, she asks? Sam tells her about the work of Professor Andrée le May.

Chapter 6   **Sourcing the best evidence**

Paul Boagy, Pat Maier and Alan Glasper
University of Southampton, UK

This chapter of the book outlines the process of finding the best evidence through an effective literature search and by making the fullest use of all the help and support provided by your university library service.

Scenario

Sue and Sam are making a plan of action that includes gathering material for their dissertation. Sue knows that quite a lot of changes have gone on in the nursing section of the library since she last used it. Sam is used to accessing some information on the Internet but is unsure of the best way of finding information on a particular topic that comes up to the right academic standards to use in his dissertation. They decide the best way to equip themselves is by consulting their university nursing librarian and asking for some tips on what they should do if they are to collect good quality articles for their dissertations.

Exploring and refining your question

As you can imagine, you cannot simply sit down in front of your computer, or stand in the library and start searching. You need to do a lot of important preparation first. So, before you start searching for papers and books you need to:
- Identify the topic of your research.
- Identify the approach you are going to take.
- Refine your question in order to target your research.
- Identify key search words or phrases.

How to Write Your Nursing Dissertation, First Edition. Alan Glasper and Colin Rees.
© 2013 John Wiley & Sons, Ltd. Published 2013 by John Wiley & Sons, Ltd.

Identifying your topic

This is easy if you have a passion for something, but be careful that you clearly identify which part of a passionate topic you want to investigate. Always check that you will be able to find enough material on the topic. One area you can check is the NHS Evidence database (http://www.evidence.nhs.uk/). On this database you can search a topic, like 'heart attack', and find relevant articles related to this topic under: diagnosis, economics, aetiology, prognosis, symptoms or therapy. Immediately you can see that saying that you want to do some research on 'heart attacks' means you need to refine it further.

Identify the approach you are going to take

Before you can start searching for your topic, you need to clearly understand what you are looking for within that topic. Some ways of looking at your topic are:

- **The Road Map approach**
  This traces the history of the topic and your work reviews its history. You will also have some critical reflection on what you review. You may want to investigate how patients with heart attacks have been treated over the last twenty years and what influenced the changes in approach and the prognosis.
- **Here we go again**
  This relates to people who are carrying out a research dissertation that includes gathering data, which many of you will not be doing. It involves the researcher using current knowledge and/or existing methodology and attempts to replicate, verify or refute previous results. They then discuss their results in light of previous work.
- **Can I prove it?**
  This is an experimental approach, again in research data gathering dissertations, where the researcher sets up a hypothesis and attempt to disprove it. This approach may be linked to the 'Here we go again' approach.
- **The Swiss Cheese approach**
  You present current knowledge where the purpose is to show where there are gaps or holes in the field that require further attention or consideration.
- **Eye-ball switch**
  You look at existing research in the light of a new approach/theory. How can you re-interpret previous research with this new lens? You may want to look at therapies, diagnosis or symptoms that have been used in the past in the light of new knowledge, or apply a technique used in one clinical setting to another where it has not currently been considered.

Take a closer look at the approaches above and identify the approach that resembles yours the most. If it is not there, then write your own approach.

Refine your research question

Once you have decided on the precise nature of your topic and the kind of approach you want to take, you can then ensure that your questions is fully refined to enable targeted searching. What aspect will you look at, for example: diagnosis, economics, aetiology, prognosis, symptoms or therapy? Is there anything else not on this list?

My aspect will be:

Sue and Sam are beginning to refine their area of study

If you are dealing with patients, can you further refine this and determine the scope of the patients you will deal with, for example: gender, age, part of the country, those having undergone a particular intervention at a particular time? Is there anything else not on this list?

The scope of the patients will be:

NB: Chapter 9 provides more detail on how to pose evidence-based practice questions.

If you are not dealing with patients, what are you dealing with, for example: hospital practice of a topic in a particular area, government policy, interprofessional working practices, and nursing attitudes? Do you want to limit the scope by identifying a particular clinical area, group of nurses? What else can you add to this list that applies to you?

I will be looking at:

Identify search words

Now you have refined your topic and its scope, you need to identify the search words that you will want to use in order to find appropriate research. Try to be as methodical as you can with this and remember that, when you do come to search, you will need to take into account the variations in certain words, for example:

- Use a related word to the one you have written down (a thesaurus might help). You want to look for synonyms.
- Consider variations in the word, for example noun, adjective, singular or plural (see 'truncation' and 'wildcard' later).
- Try using both American and UK spelling.
- Limit your phrase length in order to keep on target (only include key words in your phrase – it need not be grammatically correct).

Being aware of this is very important as you could miss some key references if you are not careful. You need to develop a method for identifying your key words; two ways of going about this are mentioned here. You may also develop your own way.

Using a mind map to identify your key words

One way is to produce a mind map either using mapping software (e.g. Mind Manager or Inspiration) or a large sheet of paper. Write the question in the centre of the paper, and then fill the rest of the sheet with as many other words, phrases, acronyms and so on as you can think of which relate to some aspect of the question. These words and phrases can then be grouped by using different coloured pens. Select one word or phrase on the sheet and mark it with one colour. Using the same colour pen, mark any other words or phrases that are related to this aspect of the question. Then select a second colour, choose an unmarked word or phrase on the sheet and repeat the process. If there are any remaining unmarked words and phrases, choose another colour and continue as before.

Using a linear figure to identify your key words

You can treat your question as a linear rectangle, divided into perhaps three or four sections, each section representing one aspect of the question. Taking each section in turn, list below it as many words or phrases as you can think of which relate to that aspect of the question.

Developing a methodical process will ensure that you systematically derive lists of key words and phrases that you can then use in your literature search. It will also give you something to return to if you need to revise your search strategy later on. The next step is to select the appropriate bibliographic databases for searching.

Searching for research articles

As part of a comprehensive search for evidence, you will need to undertake a thorough literature review. This involves identifying and evaluating the research journal articles which have been published on your topic. For this purpose you will need to have access to a range of bibliographic databases, such as CINAHL, British Nursing Index (BNI) or SCOPUS. Random browsing of the journals you happen to be aware of, or have been told about by colleagues, will help but will not be a sufficiently robust way of literature searching.

What are bibliographic databases?

Bibliographical databases are computer-based resources that provide references to the published journal literature and enable you to undertake comprehensive and systematic literature searches. Access to, and use of, these bibliographical databases assumes that you have the appropriate level of IT skills and the confidence to undertake the searching process on your own, making use of help and support where necessary.

Why we have bibliographic databases

Within their individual scope they offer a means of systematically identifying the journal and other types of literature that have been published in particular subject areas. Information on some of the most important databases covering the healthcare fields follows later.

Scenario

Sue and Sam have attended a lecture given by one of the librarians on how to search the literature. The librarian had made them laugh by describing libraries as being like the Albert Hall full from top to bottom with journal papers. Students cannot simply dive in and look for the only four papers ever published on the subject of larvae therapy for the treatment of foot wounds, as the chance of success would be statistically very small. What is needed to succeed, the students were informed, was to be systematic and use the university databases wisely.

The function of bibliographic databases

Bibliographic databases provide references to articles published in journals and, in some cases, they also cover other types of literature, such as theses and dissertations, books and book chapters, government reports and policy documents. Updated on a regular basis, the databases are searchable in different ways and provide sophisticated techniques for developing and revising your searches. Some database providers offer the facility for you to store your searches on the system, enabling you to revisit and update your literature searching as your work progresses. In some cases, current awareness services are also available for you to make use of. These services will provide automatic email alerts for you when new references that relate to your stored searches are added to the database.

Tip: If you do not know what current awareness services look like search for 'Current Contents/OVID' or simply search more generically for 'Current Awareness Services'. You may want to add 'Nursing' or 'Medical' to target your search.

How do the databases work?

The databases work by providing searching facilities to produce a list of references that can then be followed up. It is possible to search the databases in different ways – by subject keyword or phrase, author or title for example, or combinations of these. It is also possible to refine and restrict your search in a number of ways: by date of publication, type of publication, language or place of publication, for example, depending upon the facilities offered by the particular database you are using.

A search will generate a list of articles that can then be stored, downloaded or printed off from the database. In some cases a list of the cited references may be available as part of the article record. This can be a useful way of finding further references on the topic in the early stages of your searching, as well as for triangulating your search methodology (i.e. cross-referencing from several search methods). The cited references are those books, articles and other resources which the authors themselves referred to while writing their article, and are usually provided as a list at the end of the article, with links from the text of the article concerned.

In the case of some bibliographic databases, direct links from the record to the full text of the article are sometimes available; if not, then your library and information service will provide access to a range of electronic and printed journals, or to document supply facilities in cases where the journal article you need is not held locally.

Getting access to the databases

Access will be provided by your library and information service, with links via their web site; for NHS staff, they are currently provided by the electronic (NHS) Health Information Resources federated search facility. A federated search facility is a search engine that simultaneously searches a multiple of databases or web resources for you. This may sometimes be referred to as a web portal in your institution. If you are currently studying with a university, you can normally expect the databases to be available for you to use both on and off campus, via the library service's web pages.

Databases available to you

Within the healthcare field, there a number of large and powerful biblio-graphic databases that are widely used by researchers. Most of them include abstracts of the articles they reference. They are:

- **Allied and Complementary Medicine Database** [AMED] is produced by the Health Care Information Service of the British Library. It is an important data-base for complementary medicine and palliative care. It is updated monthly.
- **Applied Social Sciences Index and Abstracts** [ASSIA] is an indexing and abstracting tool covering health, social services, psychology and sociology, among other subjects. It is updated monthly.
- **British Nursing Index** [BNI] indexes the most popular English-language nursing and related journals. It is updated monthly.
- **Cumulative Index to Nursing and Allied Health Literature** [CINAHL] is a comprehensive index to literature published worldwide. Over 2500 jour-nals are currently indexed and other types of material, such as American doctoral dissertations, are also included. It includes some full text links and is updated weekly.
- **EMBASE** is a major biomedical and pharmaceutical database, indexing over 3500 international journals. It is updated weekly.
- The **Health Management Information Consortium** [HMIC] database includes references derived from two different sources: the Department of Health's Library and Information Services and the King's Fund Centre Information and Library Service. It is particularly useful for searching for references on health services policy and management, and indexes books, reports and journal articles; both parts of the database provide a useful means of identifying grey literature. It is updated bimonthly.
- **MEDLINE** is produced by the National Library of Medicine in the United States and is the most important biomedical database for literature search-ing. It indexes over 3900 journals published worldwide and is updated daily.
- **PsycINFO** is the main database for searching the literature of psychology, psychiatry and related fields. It includes references from as far back as 1806 up to the present, covering journal articles, books, chapters and dissertations. It is updated weekly.

Getting help in using the databases

Most of the databases have built-in help screens available and, in some cases, links to guide leaflets that can be printed off. You can also expect your library and information service to provide online or printed guide leaflets and help sheets, and, in most cases, one-to-one help and group tutorials. If you have never used them before, these databases can sometimes appear daunting and even the experienced searcher will need to keep up with changes to them. It is always worth seeking out some help, as discussed later.

Why it is not best practice to rely on Google

Google is easy and convenient to use but will not provide such a comprehensive and systematic survey of the literature as you will be able to achieve by using one or more of the databases outlined above. It is worth emphasising that best evidence is usually found in journal articles that have been peer reviewed, that is screened before publication by experts in the field. The main databases access peer reviewed journals but Google does not discriminate in relation to the quality of evidence in this way; rather, it depends on availability rather than quality. It is, however, important to remember that the search engine Google Scholar is a very useful first stop for investigating the parameters of just what is available. Google Scholar is a citation index and may, therefore, not host the most up to date journal papers.

Devising your search strategy

Having identified the key terms and concepts that cover your research topic, and learned something of the bibliographic databases available for searching, you can then begin to devise your search strategy.

Subject searching: keyword or free text searching

A keyword or free text search means that you will be looking for every occurrence of a particular word or phrase, wherever it appears – normally in the title or abstract of the reference – within the record. This type of search is very wide and normally retrieves the largest possible number of records, but some of the references may appear less relevant to your subject. If you use this type of search, you will need to have considered all the possible synonyms for the same concept, for example *youth, teenager, adolescent* and *young adult*, and then search the databases using each of the terms.

Using a subject thesaurus

The most important databases, such as CINAHL, MEDLINE and British Nursing Index for example, include a subject thesaurus. If you perform a search on the database using this facility, it will convert a word or phrase into the suggested main indexing term. Using this, you can gather together all the references included on the database which are indexed using the same term. This can be more effective than keyword searching if there are a number of different synonyms for your particular term. Using the example above, the

CINAHL subject heading for all of these is '*Adolescence*'; it is also possible to 'focus' on this subject heading, so that you retrieve a list of articles where this term is regarded a major aspect of the articles concerned.

A search using truncation
All of the databases also offer various other searching techniques, such as truncation and the use of wildcards. Truncation means that you can perform a keyword/free text search using a term such as *assess** (with a* after the word), which looks for assess, assessed, assessing, assessment and so on, without having to search for all the different words separately.

Similarly, if you want to search for articles that contain child, children, child's, children's, childhood then searching *child** will retrieve them all. It will, however, also retrieve 'childbirth', which is something you may not want in your particular context.

A search using wildcard
A wildcard search normally uses the '?' character, where there may be another letter present, for example, *p?ediatric* which will search for both '*paediatric*' and '*pediatric*'.

A search using Boolean logic
This keyword/free text searching technique uses one of the Boolean operators AND, OR and NOT, named after the nineteenth century mathematician who devised the system of logical operations. Using the example above, you would specify: *child** NOT childbirth.

Boolean terms:

AND
   Include both search words in search
   String ANDs to include a longer list of words
   All search words then need to be in the result
OR
   Allows for at least one of the search words to appear in the result
NOT
   Excludes a word from the search, for example child* NOT childcare.

A search using phrases
Most databases provide the facility to search for a word or phrase within the title of articles, which will give a shorter but much more focused list of references. Alternatively, you may have the name of a specific author and wish to search for all the papers written by that person. This is known as field searching, the fields being each different section of the database record.

Imposing restrictions on your search

You will also need to consider any possible limits and exclusions that you wish to incorporate in your search (for example, language, date of publication, type of material, specific methodologies etc.).

- Language: Some of the literature searching databases include references to articles published globally, in many languages, and it can be very difficult to obtain translations if you are not proficient in the language concerned. You may wish to restrict your search to English-language articles only; this facility is usually provided.
- Date: You will also need to think about restricting your search by the date of publication if you wish to retrieve references published more recently or within a particular date range. The databases sometimes include references to articles published over a very long period and will not automatically do this for you, although most of them will usually display your references in reverse date order, showing the most recent publications first in the list. How far back in the literature you need to search will depend to some extent upon the nature of the topic you are working with and upon the available published literature. Otherwise there may have been a key research paper, policy document or report which changed the subsequent nature of the research on the topic and you may only want to find articles which have been published later than that.
- Type of material: If you are only searching for journal articles, you need to bear in mind that some of the databases also include references to other types of material. For example, PsycInfo includes references to books and book chapters, as well as to journal articles, and CINAHL includes references to American college and university dissertations. HMIC includes references to grey literature as well as journal articles. Grey literature is the collective term used to describe publications which originate in ways outside mainstream publication, such as academic theses, unpublished research reports, information produced for patients and so on. Depending upon the nature of your topic you may wish to include a search for this type of material.CINAHL enables you to limit your search to research articles or to evidence-based practice, for example. You need to remember, however, that the more of these specific limits you apply to a search, the fewer references you will retrieve.
- Specific methodologies: Some of the databases enable you to include restrictions as to the type of methodology used in the research, such as provided by the Clinical Queries limit on MEDLINE.

The databases will display your search history. This will list each of the terms you have searched, indicating the number of references found in each case, and enabling you to combine different terms in the history if you wish.

If your search does not find anything or finds material not relevant

If you are unhappy with the list of references provided by your database search, you will need to revise your search. If you have not found any references at all, check your spelling and typing. The databases will only search for what you have asked for! If the references seem too specific, revisit your original mind map or diagram and look for a more general term you can use instead. Alternatively, if the search results are too general, consider a more specific term and go back to the database.

Accessing journal literature

After you have done some searching, you will want to access the article itself. So how do you do that?

When you have undertaken a search of the appropriate databases for your subject, and retrieved a list of references, you need to decide which of the references you wish to follow up. Normally, where an abstract is provided as part of the record, this is sufficient to enable you to make this decision. Sometimes, however, if there is no abstract or the title of the article is unclear, you may need to read the article itself to know whether or not it is of relevance.

To trace a particular article, look at the reference's source details. This will indicate the journal in which the article was published, as well as giving you full bibliographic details (volume and/or issue number, date and pages), enabling you to trace the article.

Knowing which journals you can access

Your library and information service will provide access to journals, in a number of ways, and will enable you to check which ones are available. Access to the electronic full-text version of the journal from the library's web catalogue, or via a journal management system (such as TDNet), linked from the library's web pages, are the two most usual means of access provided by libraries.

Using the journals themselves in electronic full text on a computer, rather than in printed format, is now the accepted means of access, except for some older material and a small number of specialist titles. This changeover from print to electronic format has taken place very quickly over the last few years and is beneficial for the user in a number of ways. Among the greatest benefits are the ease of use and convenience of access, with many people now having access to the Internet at home as well as at work. This reduces the amount of time needed to visit the library taking writing materials.

In most cases, it is straightforward to print off or download a copy of the article you need. However, you must always bear in mind the limits imposed by copyright legislation, which restricts printing or photocopying of one article from an individual issue of a journal.

Because of complicated licensing requirements, university libraries can only allow access to electronic journals for their own current students and staff. University libraries, in particular, have been able to provide access to very many more electronic full-text journals than were previously available for their users in printed format, because of the way that subscriptions and access to electronic resources has been coordinated at a national level.

e-Journals

Journals now provide their articles in electronic form and once you have searched and selected an article, you will be able to download that article onto your PC providing your institution subscribes to that journal. Increasingly you will find that most of your articles will be available in this format.

Some literature searching databases include full-text links to articles from the database records. It is often better, however, to keep the two stages of the literature searching process separate, as things can sometimes get very confusing, especially if you are an inexperienced searcher and working with more than one database and search. Search for the literature first, then follow up by tracing the articles.

Printed journals

Those libraries that still retain printed journals will record their holdings in their web catalogue, or in the case of a small library service may perhaps produce a list of them. Of course, access to printed journals will usually necessitate a visit to the library itself, unless it can offer a service whereby photocopies of articles can be sent to you.

Inter-library requests

Quite often your literature searching will identify articles that have been published in journals that are not held by your library service or available to you on the computer. It is usually possible to obtain copies of these articles by using your library's inter-library request service. This is normally regarded as a special service, as significant costs may be involved, and you may find that there is a charge for using the inter-library service, or that your use of it is restricted.

The Cochrane Library

The Cochrane Library deserves its own section. It describes itself as the best single source of reliable evidence about the effects of healthcare.

Why is it so important?

As part of a search for the best evidence, it must be regarded as the most important resource for information about the effectiveness of healthcare treatments and interventions. A web-based resource, it is currently available free of charge and without the need for user registration. It is available through the Health Information Resources, and other types of library services provide links to it from their websites in support of their own users.

The Cochrane Library comprises a number of separate databases that may be searched together or individually. These are:
- Cochrane Database of Systematic Reviews (Cochrane Reviews)
- Database of Abstracts of Reviews of Effects (Other Reviews)
- Cochrane Central Register of Controlled Trials (Clinical Trials)
- Cochrane Methodology Register (Methods Studies)
- Health Technology Assessment Database (Technology Assessments)
- NHS Economic Evaluation Database (Economic Evaluations)

The Cochrane Library also includes information about the Cochrane Collaboration, which is the international organisation involved with the work of the specialist Cochrane Review Groups, Methods Groups, Fields and Centres.

What information does the Cochrane Library contain?

Each of the component databases of the Cochrane Library contains a different type of information, as follows:

(i) Cochrane Database of Systematic Reviews (Cochrane Reviews)

Cochrane systematic reviews are the 'gold standard': the highest quality of reviews of research evidence. The database currently includes over 3500 completed reviews and more than 1800 protocols, which are reviews in progress. They deal with many different research questions. In each case, within the criteria set by the Cochrane reviewers, all the published research on the topic is assessed and evaluated using the most rigorous procedures. The aim is to determine whether or not there is conclusive evidence about the effectiveness or otherwise of the particular healthcare treatment or intervention under consideration. The completed reviews may subsequently be updated, or have comments added to them, or, in some cases, they may be withdrawn as the review becomes out of date. Any such amendments are clearly indicated in the review. For this reason, it is necessary to make a note of the particular edition of the Cochrane Library you searched. It is currently updated four times a year, and the latest edition is indicated on the main screen, with some of the new content listed. The list of reviews can be browsed in several different ways.

(ii) Database of Abstracts of Reviews of Effects (Other Reviews)
This database is produced by the Centre for Reviews and Dissemination at
the University of York. It includes structured abstracts of quality assessed
reviews of research evidence from published journal literature; newly added
abstracts are indicated. There are currently more than 5000 abstracts in this
database.

(iii) Cochrane Central Register of Controlled Trials (Clinical Trials)
Next in the hierarchy of evidence provided by the Cochrane Library, this
database includes references to randomised controlled trials, which have
been published in the research journal literature. The records are largely
derived from the EMBASE and MEDLINE bibliographical databases.
The individual references include abstracts but no links to the full text of the
journal articles concerned. There is also material in the database which is
provided by the Cochrane Review Groups themselves. The database contains
approximately 500 000 records in total.

(iv) Cochrane Methodology Register (Methods Studies)
This specialist section of the Cochrane Library deals with the methodology
of controlled trails and systematic reviews, and is produced on behalf of the
Cochrane Methodology Review Group by the UK Cochrane Centre, which is
currently part of the NHS R&D Programme, based in Oxford. It includes
references to books, journal articles and conference proceedings.

(v) Health Technology Assessment Database (Technology Assessments)
This database is produced by the Centre for Reviews and Dissemination.
It brings together details of completed and continuing health technology
assessments from around the world. It differs from the other sections of the
Cochrane Library described above in that the abstracts it contains are
descriptive rather than analytical.

(vi) NHS Economic Evaluation Database (Economic Evaluations)
The cost effectiveness of health interventions and treatments is the focus of
this part of the Cochrane Library. It is another product of the Centre for
Reviews and Dissemination, and contains over 5000 references to quality-
assessed economic evaluations.

Searching the Cochrane Library
The content of the Cochrane Library may be searched in a number of different
ways. The individual databases can be searched separately or together. On the
main page of the Cochrane Library there is a box for a basic search term, which

will search for the term in titles, abstracts and keywords across the content of all the individual databases. This works well for a very specific concept, or a named drug, for example, but is ineffective for very general words, such as 'pain' for example. Advanced searching allows more detailed searching within record titles, for example, and on-screen help is available. MeSH searching is a third option and involves the use of a thesaurus of subject headings. This facility is also available on the MEDLINE database. More information about this technique is available on screens within the Cochrane Library.

Browsing the Cochrane Library

As an alternative to the searching techniques described above, it is also possible to browse some of the individual databases within the Cochrane Library.

The Database of Systematic Reviews can be browsed in several ways:

- Topic
- New Reviews and Protocols
- Updated reviews
- An A-Z list
- Cochrane Review Group.

The Cochrane Methodology Register (Methods Studies), the Health Technology Assessment Database (Technology Assessments) and the NHS Economic Evaluation Database (Economic Evaluations) may all be browsed alphabetically, with newly added entries indicated through the list. The Database of Abstracts of Reviews of Effects (Other Reviews) and the Cochrane Central Register of Controlled Trials (Clinical Trials) are both deemed too large to facilitate browsing, and advanced searching is offered as an alternative.

Getting help using the Cochrane Library

The Cochrane Library provides a comprehensive assortment of support information targeted at different user groups. There are links to this material from the main page, and it may be downloaded. There is information here for the new user as well as for the expert researcher. It is also worth asking your library service if they have produced a guide leaflet. If they have, then it is likely to be written in a way they know will assist their clients.

Websites and other resources

The Internet has now become the accepted way for many people beginning a search for information. Access to the Internet at home, as well at work, or using the local public library, or university or college networks, is now a reality, and it is possible to have access to knowledge on a global scale.

The amount of accessible information can be bewildering, if not overwhelming, and you need to be able to navigate your way through it all. In particular, you need to be able to distinguish the good from the bad (or downright misleading, or even dangerous). Great care must be taken to ensure that you only use information from quality assured, authoritative and up-to-date sites.

Evaluation of websites

One of the most important websites currently available to you is the Health Information Resources, which is a comprehensive electronic library and information service provided for the National Health Service. This encompasses a very wide range of information resources, guidance and specialist advice tailored for the health practitioner. It includes direct links to other evidence-based resources, such as the Cochrane Library, as well as to sources of clinical guidance and of images, and also to some of the bibliographic databases discussed earlier. As the working library for the National Health Service, it also provides password-controlled access to a range of electronic journals, electronic books and databases. It is searchable in a number of different ways and detailed online assistance is provided.

Important features of the Health Information Resources are the specialist libraries, which gather together the resources within a number of major clinical areas, such as cancer, diabetes, and stroke, for example, as well as some generic areas, such as women's health and child health. The search facility within each of the specialist libraries encompasses not only evidence and guidance but also some types of grey literature, such as reports and policy documents, learning materials, information on organisations, conferences and courses, as well as patient-related information.

The specialist libraries also offer an effective way of keeping up-to-date with new material as it becomes available, with current awareness and alerting services.

Support from your library service

If you are currently working in the National Health Service, or are studying at a university or college, you will have access to a library and information service, which perhaps you may not have used very much in the past. The library has a crucial part to play in supporting your dissertation work by providing the resources and facilities you will need.

There are a number of different types of library:
- Those provided by National Health Service Trusts.
- Academic libraries, provided by universities and colleges.

- Public libraries.
- Information services in other types of organisation, which may be provided by an information specialist working as part of a multiprofessional team.
- Libraries provided by professional organisations such as the Royal College of Nursing (RCN).
- Charitable trusts and foundations, such as the King's Fund Centre.

The way the library and information service is delivered will differ in some respects in each case, for example regarding the amount of individual assistance it is possible to provide for users and the availability of library resources.

You may be able to access a number of different library services, across different sectors, depending upon your circumstances at the time, as long as you conform to the membership requirements of the particular library. On the other hand, you may find it more convenient and beneficial to use one particular library, and to develop a close relationship with the service and with the staff who can assist you.

If you currently work in the NHS, you can find details of your local NHS library by searching the Health Library and Information Services Directory website (http://www.hlisd.org/, *last accessed 10 August 2010*). This currently provides details of more than 900 library and information services, and is searchable by library or staff name, or geographically by place or postcode.

The assistance you will receive from your library/information service will include:

- Making available a selection of text books, to enable you to read around your research topic for background information.
- Providing printed journals, reports, official documents, DVDs/videos and other types of material, as well as access to electronic information resources such as databases and journals via the Internet.
- Helping and advising with all stages of the literature searching process and document delivery.
- Training in Information skills – on a one-to-one basis, and in groups.
- Updating you on changes to information resources and services.
- Providing face-to-face, email and web-based enquiry services.
- Providing an inter-library services for you with books and journal articles not held locally.
- Accessing detailed information via the library service's web pages.
- Trouble shooting, when you are really stuck!

Each type of library strives to provide an efficient and effective service within the scope of its available resources. Now is the time to get to know your library and make the most of what it has to offer.

RCN information literacy competencies

> **Scenario**
>
> Sue and Sam have found their local librarians to be a huge asset in helping them understand the complexities of searching the literature and have found information from the Royal College of Nursing very helpful.

Additionally, the RCN has developed literacy competences to help nurses bolster evidence-based practice and has launched a strategy to help nurses and other health care professionals deliver and improve evidence-based practice (EBP)(http://www.rcn.org.uk/__data/assets/pdf_file/0007/357019/003847.pdf).

> **Activity**
>
> The RCN has made its full strategy available to readers of this book.
> Go to the companion website of this book at www.wiley.com/go/glasper/ nursingdissertation and download the competencies.

The College has recognised that nurses need to develop information literacy competencies to boost their skills in harnessing information from a wide range of sources to make a difference to their delivery of safe and effective care based on best available evidence. Their initiative has a clear mission of supporting an individual practitioner's abilities to source, interpret and synthesise information for the ultimate benefit to patient care. The RCN plans to underpin this initiative with a range of on-line resources to show how nurses can use the new competencies in their day-to-day caring activities. These competencies have been influenced by similar work conducted in Australia and New Zealand (www.caul.edu.au).

The quest for the delivery of evidence-based nursing care underpins the whole stance of the Nursing and Midwifery Council's decision to legislate for the introduction of new degree level standards to underpin pre-registration nursing education which commenced in 2011.

Graduate education is assumed to help nurses develop the skill of finding and applying evidence to improve and therefore change practice. However, it is not always recognised that a major key to evidence-based practice is the ability to process information. In particular, much depends on the wording of a clear patient outcome question that will produce search terms for an effective review of the literature. This will generate appropriate articles that can then be critiqued and synthesised and a decision made on whether the solution indicated by the literature should be used to change local practice. The RCN strategy on information literacy was, therefore, aimed to help guide nurses in developing information processing skills that would benefit those in their care.

What are the RCN information literacy competencies?

These competencies are primarily designed to help nurses evaluate professional standards and bench marks. UNESCO (2009) believes that people who are information literate are better able to use information to make informed judgements. The NMC clearly recognises this, as it has, within its new standards for pre-registration education, made it clear that it wants tomorrow's nurse to be able to develop skills to find, manage and evaluate information, and apply that information and evidence to their day-to-day activities as carers.

The RCN have identified seven discrete areas of information literacy competence which are intended to be used as a framework to support nurses and nursing teams to use information wisely.

1 *Identifying why information is needed*

Nurses need to understand why information is needed and to pose a question which can be answered through a critical analysis of the literature to identify gaps between current knowledge and new knowledge, with the aim of new ideas for care delivery. To achieve this, nurses need to develop skills in identifying, sorting, classifying and using key words and terms.

2 *Identifying what information is needed*

Here nurses should be able to position the topic area within their care parameters, be able to identify limits and use relevant primary and secondary sources of information. This requires nurses who are skilled at using information from across inter-professional boundaries, being able navigate a library and to use a range of scholarly databases. Importantly, nurses will need to be able to weigh up the strength of the evidence they liberate after critical appraisal of the information and make judgements accordingly (Greenhalgh, 2001). The ability of nurses to able to critically appraise a variety of types of evidence is crucial to the RCN strategy, which demands professionals who can critically appraise the evidence and make judgements about its rigour and transferability to the clinical practice setting.

3 *Carrying out a search to find information*

To be able to achieve any of these competencies nurses need to identify where relevant information can be found. This requires an ability not only to navigate and use a library and interrogate databases but also to know the good from the bad and the ugly. Hence, nurses need to learn to use trustworthy sources of information and to be able to use inclusion and excision criteria to avoid being swamped with information. It is the judicious use of literature search terms and strategies which prevents nurses from 'diving into the Albert Hall filled with tens of thousands of journal papers' with the expectation of finding the one paper dealing with the efficacy of larvae therapy on wound healing.

To avoid this nurses have to learn to manage information in such a way as to use key words and terms to focus their searching activities. This can be made easier by the use of truncation, wild cards and Boolean logic. By learning to use inclusion and exclusion criteria irrelevant information can be filtered out. In using online collections, such as Internurse, full-text papers can be retrieved for greater scrutiny (http://www.internurse.com/cgi-bin/go.pl/library/index.html). Internurse is one of the UK's largest online archive of peer-reviewed nursing articles and is home to over 9000 peer reviewed articles from 14 key health journals; this and other similar archives can help nurses keep abreast of innovations in EBP (Gerrish *et al.*, 2004). Additionally, nurses need to be able to use data from clinical audit and expert opinions from colleagues to reinforce the findings they retrieve from literature.

4 *Evaluating how the information meets the identified need*
Crucial to EBP is the ability of the nurse to make judgments of the relevance of the information sourced. In this situation it is necessary to check for any deficits in the information by using a critical appraisal tool. For example, The Critical Appraisal Skills Programme (CASP) suite of critiquing tools was designed originally by McMaster University in Canada to help healthcare professionals make sense of the evidence they found in scholarly journal articles (http://www.sph.nhs.uk/what-we-do/public-health-workforce/resources/critical-appraisals-skills-programme).

Such tools, of which there are many, help nurses check for bias in the published work and help them make a judgement of the worth of the evidence overall and whether it merits further investigation before a change is warranted in practice. Hence, nurses need to develop competencies to allow them to judge if the information they are reading is accurate, reliable and valid. They also need to make judgments about the source of the information they have retrieved and recognise both the strengths and limitations of knowledge-sharing discussion groups, such as wikis and blogs, being able to recognise bias and cultural contexts.

5 *Using information and knowledge inclusively, legally and ethically*
The RCN competency framework expects nurses to be able to seek information that is inclusive and culturally sensitive. All appropriate evidence where and when warranted should be used to underpin practice and make changes where necessary. Importantly, the new framework highlights the

dangers of plagiarism and the necessity of having knowledge about the storage of information and how that information is communicate to others. In a tabloid world where breaches of confidentiality appear on a regular basis, nurses need to be aware of the importance of information security, especially where patient data are involved. Thus, Caldicott principles are pivotal to the RCN strategy (http://www.dh.gov.uk/en/ Publicationsandstatistics/Publications/PublicationsPolicyAndGuidance/ DH_4068403).

6   *Managing information*
Perhaps one of the most important aspects of the RCN strategy is the emphasis on nurses being able to create a scholarly audit trail, where the provenance of their information seeking, note taking and reference recoding for future retrieval of literature is transparent and replicable. All of this requires diligence in developing systems for organising and managing information. There are now a range of software tools available to help professionals manage their EBP bibliographies (e.g. http://www.refman.com/).

The ability of professionals to network with fellow colleagues around the UK and further afield is embraced by the RCN, which advocates for nurses to actively subscribe to discussion groups and organisations such as the Association of Chief Children's Nurses (ACCN) (http://www. accnuk.org). Such organisations are invaluable in promoting EBP.

7   *Creating new information or knowledge*
The final aspect of the RCN strategy for promoting EBP encourages nurses to draw conclusions from the knowledge bases they have appraised and to recognise that a lack of information can also be classed as evidence. Importantly, the whole thrust of the strategy is for nurses to harness evidence as a positive prompt for change and improvements in practice where key messages of research can be translated into action. Finding the evidence to support a change in practice requires knowledge of how to act as a change agent and, furthermore, disseminating that evidence to others. This requires nurses who are able to write summative reports which are convincing and authoritative. Nurses who can articulate their EBP findings to others through journal publications, conference presentations and poster presentations are well placed to promote excellence in patient care.

Conclusion

The process of EBP can be summarised as:
- Asking a question.
- Finding evidence.
- Appraising the evidence.

- Making judgements.
- Making recommendations.

Healthcare professionals with these skills will be needed in the future and will be of enormous help in meeting the aspirations of all the health professions in their quest to deliver care based on best evidence.

Scenario

Sue and Sam feel ready to commence their search of the databases.

References

Gerrish, K., Entwistle, B., Parmakis, G. *et al.* (2004) Sharing best practice. *Developing a web based data base. British Journal of Nursing,* **13** (1), 44–48.

Greenhalgh, T. (2001) *How to read a paper the basis of evidence based medicine.* BMJ Publishing Group, London.

UNESCO (2009) *Information Literacy.* UNESCO, Paris (available from: http://portal. unesco.org/ci/en/ev.php-URL_ID=27055&URL_DO=DO_TOPIC&URL_ SECTION=201.html; accessed 23 January 2011).

For further resources for this chapter visit the companion website at

🖱 **www.wiley.com/go/glasper/nursingdissertation**

Chapter 7 What is grey literature and where can it be found?

Alan Glasper[1] and Colin Rees[2]
[1]University of Southampton, UK
[2]University of Cardiff, UK

Scenario

Sam and Sue have been asked by their supervisors to ensure that all aspects of grey literature have been explored and reflected in their literature review. Sue is not at all clear how to identify 'grey literature' and is concerned that she may miss a vital component to her literature search.

All students completing evidence-based practice dissertations need to fully appraise any grey literature pertinent to their field of study. The Internet is now the largest source for the identification of grey literature.

What is 'grey literature'?

Firstly, grey literature is not grey! It comes in a variety of colours and sizes, some good, some bad and some just ugly. Grey literature is mainly composed of any literature that is not formally published in usual publishing formats such as text books or journal articles.

The term grey literature refers primarily to papers, reports or other documents produced and published by, for example, Strategic Health Authorities, NHS Trusts, Governmental agencies, universities and other groups such as the NMC. These publications are not produced commercially, as in text books or journals, by well-known publishers and will, therefore, not have an ISBN (International Standard Book Number) or similar indexing. Although the Internet has made a huge difference to how grey literature is sourced many of these documents can be difficult to obtain. For example, many PhD theses have to be borrowed from individual university libraries. Significant contributions to the body of grey literature are translations from foreign language published papers.

How to Write Your Nursing Dissertation, First Edition. Alan Glasper and Colin Rees.
© 2013 John Wiley & Sons, Ltd. Published 2013 by John Wiley & Sons, Ltd.

Importantly, Alberani *et al.* (1990) have explored the importance of grey literature as a means of primary but non-conventionally published communication. It is important to stress that these bodies of literature, which are often original and of recent origin, cannot always be found easily through conventional channels.

Where can I find grey literature?

There are many websites that can help in locating and exploring the useful body of information contained in grey literature. Importantly, the World Wide Web has become the portal for grey literature in the twenty-first century.

The Healthcare Management Information Consortium (HMIC) database contains records from the Library and Information Services department of the Department of Health (DH) in England and the King's Fund Information and Library Service. These combined databases are considered to be a good source of grey literature on topics such as health and community care management, organisational development, inequalities in health, user involvement, and race and health.

DH Data is the database of the Department of Health's Library and Information Services and contains in excess of 174 000 records relating to health and social care management information. Coverage includes official publications, journal articles and grey literature on: health service policy, management and administration, with an emphasis on the British National Health Service; the quality of health services including hospitals, nursing, primary care and public health; the planning, design, construction and maintenance of health service buildings; occupational health; control and regulation of medicines; medical equipment and supplies; and social care and personal social services. It includes all DH publications, including circulars and press releases. The majority of records are from 1983 onwards, although coverage of departmental materials dates back to 1919. Over a quarter of the records have abstracts.

The King's Fund is an independent health charity that works to develop and improve management of health and social care services. The King's Fund Information and Library Service database holds records of the material in the library of the King's Fund Information and Library Service. The database contains over 70 000 records (1979 to date).

This Health Management and Policy Database, from The Healthcare Management Information Consortium (HMIC), is an invaluable source of information for healthcare administrators and managers.

Important websites

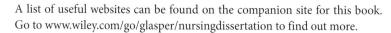

A list of useful websites can be found on the companion site for this book. Go to www.wiley.com/go/glasper/nursingdissertation to find out more.

What about Google scholar?

> **Scenario**
>
> Sam and Sue have been asked by one of their fellow students if they can use Google Scholar as a short-cut to finding published and unpublished papers.

Jasco (2008) has highlighted the pros and cons of using Google Scholar to conduct comprehensive literature search. Although Google Scholar is essentially a citation index, in other words papers have to be cited by other authors before they appear on the site, it is a useful resource. Despite the weaknesses, Google Scholar enables users to search specifically for a wide range of scholarly literature.

References

Alberani, V., Pietrangeli, P. and Mazza, M.R. (1990) The use of grey literature in health sciences: a preliminary survey. *Bulletin of the Medical Library Association*, **78** (4), 358–362.

Jacso, P. (2008) The pros and cons of computing the h-index using Google Scholar. *Online Information Review*, **32** (3), 437–452.

For further resources for this chapter visit the companion website at
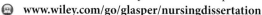 **www.wiley.com/go/glasper/nursingdissertation**

Chapter 8 Harvard or Vancouver – getting it right all the time

Alan Glasper[1] and Colin Rees[2]
[1]*University of Southampton, UK*
[2]*University of Cardiff*, UK

Scenario

Sue and Sam have been instructed by their university faculty office to use the Harvard reference system. They have been informed that reference errors carry a 10% marking penalty. Sue, who is conscious of her lower grades as a diploma student, always found referencing difficult but she does not want to lose marks at this stage and thus jeopardise her eventual honours classification.

An important aspect of your dissertation is referencing the authors you have used throughout your work. This is part of academic work where you are expected to provide evidence or support for the major statements you make and to the arguments you include in the dissertation. They are also required to avoid plagiarism, in that the words and ideas of others must be acknowledged in your work and must not be presented as if they are your own ideas. It is worth making the distinction between 'references', which includes all the authors whose work you have mentioned or 'referred' to in your dissertation, and 'bibliography', which includes work you may have read and found useful background work but is not directly referred to in your work. Many institutions do not require bibliographies, as there is no real evidence you have read them and so they may be not be relevant.

References should be key to the topic and, as far as possible, be recent. The way you show whose work you have included can take a number of different forms. In this section, we will consider two of the main referencing systems. The aim of this section is to consider the basic principles of referencing and illustrate the key features of the Vancouver and Harvard methods.

How to Write Your Nursing Dissertation, First Edition. Alan Glasper and Colin Rees.
© 2013 John Wiley & Sons, Ltd. Published 2013 by John Wiley & Sons, Ltd.

Referencing is an aspect of academic work that many people have found not difficult but irksome, as it is often responsible for some negative feedback comments on assignments. Yet by following some basic principles it is possible to avoid losing 'easy marks'.

Scenario

Sue and Sam are talking over coffee. Sue asks Sam if he has problems with referencing as, no matter how much she tries, she always seems to lose marks and get comments about the standard of her referencing. Sam agrees it is something that has frequently frustrated him. They both decide to avoid losing important marks in their dissertations by having a session together to improve their referencing skills.

The form of referencing you use should be the one 'approved' by your institution. This will be stated in your course or programme handbook. As there are variations to the two systems we show you, it is recommended that you use both the system and variation suggested by your institution. This may require you to 'translate' some references that you might encounter into your 'approved' system.

Referencing systems relate to how you indicate a source of your reading in two parts of your work or dissertation, these are: (i) in the body of your work and (ii) in the list of references at the end of your work. While the list is not usually included in your word count, those in the body are, so it is important to take this into account where you want to remain inside the word limit for your work.

Vancouver system

This system is not frequently used in UK universities but is frequently found in medical journals, so it is worth knowing how it works. It works using a number system for each source instead of using the name of the author or authors of a publication. It takes its name from a meeting of medical journal editors in Vancouver, Canada, in 1978. The problem for journals is how to make best use of space, so it was decided that those publishing in medical journals should allocate a number to each reference in turn and then list them in number order at the end. This would also help the flow of the article for the reader. The names of the journals were also abbreviated in the reference list to save more space. The numbers in the main body of a work are in brackets as close to the point made as possible, such as 'this has been shown in the work by Harrow (1) who found…'. This is useful for students, as it is

Table 8.1   The Vancouver system.

Source to be used	How it would look in the references section
Book	1. Kent C *Superbugs And Their Impact on Healthcare*. 3 ed. Cardiff: Kimberly Press. 2012
Chapter in a book	2. Parker P The role of the nurse in supporting patients with arachnophobia. In: Allen B (ed.) *Fast Acting Treatments for Phobias and Anxiety States*. 3rd ed. Oxford: University Press. 2012. P32–44.
Journal	3. Wayne B and Grayson D Evidence-based practice and larvae therapy in wound care. *BJN*. 2012; 34 (5): 25–29.
Web-based reference	4. Prince D. Wonder and amazement; the lived experience of women caring for a child with chronic illness. *Qual Res Nurs*. 2012. (accessed 29/11/2012)

(Each reference is preceded by a number indicating its numeric sequence within the body of the work. This list assumes that the examples above appeared in sequence.)

easy to type a number in brackets. Each time the same work is mentioned the original number is used again, so in the example above the work by Harrow would be (1) each time it was used. Where there are several authors you want to mention in relation to one point and they have already mentioned, if they are in order you can indicate this as follows: 'several authors have been seen to favour this method of assessment (3–6, 8, 10).'

Where you need to use a page number, this can be shown as follows, 'according to Harrow (1 p.6)…'. In journals the author number is used in a more elaborate way by using a 'superscript' number, that is above the line, as in 'this has been shown in the work by Harrow[1] who found…'. Page numbers are then showed like this: 'according to Harrow [1(p.6)]…' Table 8.1 shows some of the main features of the system. A number of versions are used, so always check which you are encouraged to use.

Harvard system

This has been in use a great deal longer than the Vancouver system and is adopted as the recommended style by many Universities and nursing journals. There are a number of variations to this too, so care has to be taken to always follow the version approved by your institution. Instead of numbers this uses the authors name and year of publication as the main identifiers in the main body of work. In the reference section the references are presented in alphabetical order and are not numbered or listed in the order in which they appear in the main body. Journal names are used in full. In the body of the work, the author's name and year are used in a number of different ways.

As the subject of the sentence:

i) In the study by Johns (2012) it was shown…'
   Both Michael (2011) and Johns (2012) agree…'

Where the author provides the idea for the statement:

However, several authors have disagreed with this method (Michael 2011, Johns 2012).

In the last example both the author's name and year of publication are in brackets as they indicate the source of the information or point.

Where there are several authors of a single reference it is usual, if there are three or more names, to just use the first name in the body of your work followed by 'et al' and the year, where 'et al' means 'with others'. For example, 'Owen et al (2011) found several examples…' In the references section all the names are usually shown. However, as it has become increasingly popular for a large number of authors to be involved in publishing a single article, some referencing systems suggest that if there are six or more authors to list the first three followed by 'et al'.

There are some examples that need explanation, such as where an author is mentioned by a further author and you want to use the first author's point:

Werther (2]009) cited in Hauxwell (2011) believed that …'

In this example, only Hauxwell would appear in the reference section, as you have not read Werther's original work and the rule of referencing is that it is where you have read the work that must be indicated to the reader. This also applies to the Vancouver system.

The second difficulty often encountered is where the work is related to the author of a chapter in a book edited by someone else. In the main body you use the authors' name and year the edited book was published as usual but in the references section it is shown as indicated in Table 8.2.

Notice that book titles and journal names are in italics and, unlike the Vancouver system, the title of the journal appears in full. The abbreviation for edition is 'edn.' here, unlike the Vancouver system that uses 'ed' for both editor and edition depending on the context. You only need to show the edition number for second and subsequent editions; a first edition is not indicated.

Both approaches to referencing illustrated in this section follow a similar goal of providing a systematic and consistent approach to listing the

Table 8.2 The Harvard system.

Source to be used	How it would look in the references section
Book	Kent C (2012) *Superbugs And Their Impact on Healthcare.* (3rd edn.). Cardiff: Kimberly Press.
Chapter in a book	Parker P (2012) The role of the nurse in supporting patients with arachnophobia. In: Allen B (ed.) *Speedy Treatments for Phobias and Anxiety States.* Cardiff: Kimberly Press.
Journal	Wayne B and Grayson D (2012) The advantages of larvae therapy in wound care. *British Journal of Nursing.* 34 (5) 25–29.
Web-based reference	Prince D (2012) Wonder and amazement; the lived experience of women caring for a child with chronic illness. *Qualitative Research in Nursing.* http://www. qualitativeresearchinnursing.oxfordjournals.com/contents/ pdf/6943-312-3-42.pdf (accessed 29/11/2012).

NB: This is not how they would appear in the references section as they would appear in alphabetical order.

elements of a source of evidence. These will allow the reader to locate the information you used in your dissertation. Although similar elements are included, the order of the elements and the amount of detail does vary, so it is important not to confuse them and combine elements from both systems.

Use of computer referencing packages

There are a number of computer packages, such as Endnote©, that can be purchased or obtained through your institution that will help put your references order. These will allow you to enter the details for a reference and then provide it in a number of different formats. As always, the advice is that you should ensure that the result conforms that the system approved by your institution.

You will use many references in the course of developing your dissertation. One of the biggest tips is to start the references section when you start writing your first draft. The first time you include a reference in the draft start your reference section either in a separate file or by pressing enter ten times, putting the heading 'References' and then writing the reference in full in the approved system. Each new reference should be added in the appropriate place. Once the dissertation is complete, the reference section will also be complete and will just need to be checked if any references have been added or deleted at any stage without the reference section being adjusted.

Conclusion

As the standard of your referencing says something about your attention to detail and your academic standard, it is worth ensuring that your referencing skills are high. This section should have increased your understanding of the two main systems and how to complete appropriate references for a range of sources.

For further resources for this chapter visit the companion website at
www.wiley.com/go/glasper/nursingdissertation

Chapter 9   Posing an evidence-based practice question: Using the PICO and SPICE models

Alan Glasper[1] and Colin Rees[2]
[1]*University of Southampton, UK*
[2]*University of Cardiff,* UK

Scenario

Sam has selected a likely topic for his dissertation. He wants to explore the lived experiences of families with a child with a chronic illness but wants to ensure that it is suitable for a dissertation subject. He talks to Sue about her choice, which is the use of larvae therapy for wound healing in older women with varicose leg ulcers. During a class discussion Sue has been struggling with framing her question using the PICO or SPICE Model. Their lecturers have been explicit in the need to formulate an answerable question using one of these models. They have also been instructed to pose their evidence-based practice question at the conclusion of their dissertation introductory chapter before writing the literature search chapter.

It is important to stress that the creation of a precise and answerable question in your dissertation will allow a more efficient literature search and eventual retrieval of papers. After interrogation and critical appraisal of the papers an individual will be able to come to a conclusion as to whether the answer to the question will allow a change in practice. There are a number of models designed to help in the formulation of an answerable question. Only the PICO and SPICE models are considered here.

What is the PICO model?

Straus *et al.* (2005) outlined the PICO model of formulating a focused and answerable question. There are four elements to the posing of a PICO question. These four common features of the PICO format are helpful in allowing

---

How to Write Your Nursing Dissertation, First Edition. Alan Glasper and Colin Rees.
© 2013 John Wiley & Sons, Ltd. Published 2013 by John Wiley & Sons, Ltd.

healthcare practitioners to carefully consider the questions they wish the literature they interrogate to answer. Melnyk and Fineout-Overholt (2005) believe that each aspect of the PICO format should be considered in depth to generate a clearly articulated question. The four elements are:

1 P = Population
2 I = Intervention
3 C = Control
4 O = Outcome

Booth (2006) outlines each element of the PICO model as follows:

Population – the recipients or potential beneficiaries of a service or intervention; the population can be patients or clients with, for example:

- A disease or condition (patients with gastro-intestinal disease).
- A stage of disease (patients with advanced Chrohn's disease).
- A specific gender (women with post-natal depression).
- Age group (children with Chrohn's disease).
- Socioeconomic group (semi-skilled and unskilled manual workers with alcohol-related disease).
- Healthcare setting (mental healthcare patients attending an outpatient department).

Intervention – the service or planned action that is being delivered to the population; this could be one of a number of interventions, for example:

- A type of drug therapy for renal disease, surgical procedures used in renal disease, types of radiotherapy used in treating malignancies and so on.
- A level of intervention; for example the frequency of administration of a particular medication or the dosage of a particular drug or radiotherapy treatment.
- The stage of intervention; for example this may be expressed as prevention, secondary or advanced.
- The delivery of an intervention; for example by intravenous infusion or by self-medication and so on.

Comparison – an alternative service or action that may or may not achieve similar outcomes. For example, the use of peritoneal dialysis as a comparison with haemodialysis or the use of antibiotic drug 'A' compared with antibiotic drug 'B'. In some cases the comparison may be the usual named interventions or no intervention.

Outcomes – the ways in which the service or action can be measured to establish whether or not it has had a desired effect. This can be expressed as what happened to the population being studied as a direct result of the intervention. This can be expressed in a number of ways:

- It might be specifically patient oriented, as in an improvement in quality of life, a reduction in the severity of their symptoms or a reduction in adverse events such as drug errors. However, these should be expressed in measurable ways such as 'lower pain scores', 'fewer episodes of nausea and vomiting', anything that shows there has been a clear and measurable difference as a result of the intervention.

- It might also be organisation orientated, such as cost effectiveness, less days in hospital or a reduction in the number of personal injury claims or complaints by patients.

In this way, Huang *et al.* (2006) have suggested that the use of the mnemonic PICO helps practitioners to more precisely pose a clinically-related question in trying to answer a perceived clinical problem. Additionally, using the PICO framework will result in improved literature search strategies using the words in the PICO statement as the key search terms in the databases. This will generate more accurate results that are more likely to locate data driven papers that when subjected to critical appraisal will help to provide support or rejection of the proposed intervention.

Examples of PICO formulated questions

> *This section is designed to allow you an opportunity to examine a range of questions that might help you consider the formulation of your own dissertation question and search strategy key words.*

PICO question example 1 (a humorous example)

In 1999, the 23rd Annual Report of the Home Accident Surveillance System (http://www.hassandlass.org.uk/query/reports/1999.pdf) estimated that 3695 accidents in the UK involved trousers. Although the annual report does not specify what type of injury and it could be zipper related or simply caused by falling whilst removing them, first and crucially in the process of undertaking an evidence-based practice enquiry is to formulate an answerable question. Were students seriously looking to address the accident rate caused by trousers a PICO question might be formulated as:

Population – Trouser wearing men over 30 years of age.

Intervention – Replacing trousers with kilts.

Comparison – None or perhaps togas (why not as the toga movie, once the oldest of the Hollywood movie genres, is suddenly back in fashion!).

Outcome – A reduction in the number of trouser caused injuries.

PICO question example 2 (more serious)

It is very important when using PICO to formulate focussed, answerable questions. **NOT** for example:

Are febrile convulsions in babies dangerous?

In this example there is no intervention (I), comparison (C), or outcome measure (O). The answer to such a question may simply be 'yes' and so result in a very short dissertation!

Ask specific focussed and answerable questions, for example:

Does a febrile convulsion in a nine-month-old infant increase the likelihood that they will go on to have convulsions in later life?

However, this can go even further and provide a well-structured dissertation if you think about best practice and the interventions that may help reduce the rate of convulsions. So, you may improve on this by considering an intervention and comparison as in:

Population – Infants under one year of age who have suffered from a febrile convulsion.

Intervention – Treatment following UK NICE guidelines (http://www.nice.org.uk/cg047).

Comparison – The use of antipyretic medication

Outcome – A reduction in the number of convulsions in later life.

PICO question example 3

Is acupuncture effective in improving recovery from stroke?

Population – Men over 60 who have suffered a stoke.

Intervention – Acupuncture: duration of treatment, frequency and so on.

Comparison – Standard stoke rehabilitation programmes.

Outcome – Higher stroke recovery rate measured in time and scale to measure level of mobility.

PICO question example 4

Is the use of exercise more efficient than antidepressants for treating depression in women over 40 years of age?

Population – Women suffering from depression (severity? from a particular socioeconomic group? from a specific healthcare setting?).

Intervention – Exercise (what type, e.g. running? how strenuous? how often, e.g. twice daily?).

Comparison – Antidepressants medication (type? dose? frequency? and duration?).

Outcome – Lower level of depression as measured by a depression scale.

PICO question example 5

Does the use of antibiotics for middle ear infection in children fewer than five years of age reduce the incidence of mastoiditis?

Population – Preschool children with acute otitis media (socioeconomic factors? or households with ambient tobacco residue?).

Intervention – Antibiotics (which antibiotic? what dose? how frequent? which method of administration?).

Comparison – No intervention.

Outcome – Number of subsequent episodes of mastoiditis (cost effectiveness?).

PICO question example 6 (a biblical example)

In Chapter 3 we cited the first recorded clinical trial, which features in the Old Testament and which clearly shows an allocation of children to a dietary group, one group eating the royal foods and wine of the King Nebuchadnezzar, namely meat, and the other group a vegetarian diet in the form of pulses with water only. The aim of this trial was to ascertain differences in 'countenance' (usually referring to appearance but especially related to the face and how it is perceived by onlookers).

Population – Israeli children and Israeli children from the royal families (N = unknown). Inclusion criteria included: blemish free, wise, able to learn a language and with an understanding of science (remember gender was not stated!).

Intervention – A new diet consisting of the Kings meat (not stated but? lamb, chicken or possibly goat or even camel) and wine (this is not stipulated but was it red or white, what was the grape variety, was it grown on south facing vineyards and, importantly, what percentage of alcohol did it contain and how much did they drink – was it more than 28 units per week?)

Comparison – Four children including Daniel who had a diet of pulses (not stated in the Old Testament but it may have been broad beans or perhaps fava beans) and water (not stated in the Old Testament but was it still or sparkling or just well water?).

Outcome – Countenance. (Is this a valid measure of health and how is it measured? Is there a 'countenance scale' to provide a numeric value?)

Many researchers find the PICO model appropriate for a whole range of clinical questions

What is the SPICE model?

The SPICE model has been proposed by Booth (Booth and Brice, 2004) and is a derivation of the PICO model. It was designed originally for use primarily by librarians to help more clearly focus some types of literature search enquiry that did not always fit the PICO framework. The SPICE model framework has five components and is helpful for students who are not asking a clinically focused question. The mnemonic stands for:

1   **Setting** (Where and what is the context?)
2   **Perspective** (For whom? Who are users/potential users of service?)
3   **Intervention** (What is being done to them/for them?)
4   **Comparison** (Compared with what? What are alternatives?)
5   **Evaluation** (With what result and how will you measure whether the intervention will succeed?)

Although the SPICE structure is similar to that of PICO, Booth (2009) points out that by separating the traditional medical type population aspect of the PICO model into, firstly, a setting and, secondly, a perspective this enables SPICE to be used for posing non-medical type questions, that is more of a social scientific approach. Similarly, by substituting the term *outcome* with the term *evaluation* the SPICE model of posing a question facilitates other elements of research which are broader and incorporate concepts such as outputs or impacts.

SPICE question example 1

The first example below is from The Belgian Health Care Knowledge Centre (KCE). This is a semi-governmental institution which analyses healthcare data from various research studies with the aim of improving evidence-based practice.

What is the impact of an increase in the level of cost sharing on access to health services for the chronically ill in European countries?

Setting: (A selection of) European countries.

Perspective: Chronically-ill patients.

Intervention: Increased cost sharing (from among the European community).

Comparison: No increase in current finding arrangements.

Evaluation: Access to health services.

Activity

Access The Belgian Health Care Knowledge Centre (KCE) (http://www.kce.fgov.be/index_en.aspx?SGREF=5225) and investigate the various research questions hosted there using the SPICE model.

SPICE question example 2

How does it feel to wait for your relative (child, spouse/partner or parent) to return to the ward after emergency surgery and await the results?

Setting: Hospital surgical wards.

Perspective: Relatives of patients requiring emergency surgery.

Intervention: Dedicated waiting area with refreshments and tangible levels of distraction, such as flat screen televisions or contemporary topical magazines.

Comparison: No special area or levels of distraction.

Evaluation: By questionnaire given to relative when leaving the hospital or on return home.

Scenario

Sam and Sue are now much clearer on how to pose an answerable question and how this links to their search strategy for their literature reviews. They also have two clear ways in which they can structure their question depending on the nature of the question.

Activity

Go the book website at www.wiley.com/go/glasper/nursingdissertation and download the PICO and SPICE mnemonic proformas.
Practice writing answerable questions in your learning group.

References

Booth, A. (2006) Clear and present questions: formulating questions for evidence based practice. *Library Hi Tech*, **24** (3), 355–368. DOI: 10.1108/07378830610692127.

Booth, A. (2009) A Bridge Too Far? Stepping Stones For Evidence-Based Practice In An Academic Context. *New Review of Academic Librarianship*, **15**, 3–34.

Booth, A. and Brice, A. (2004) *Formulating Answerable Questions. Evidence Based Practice: An Information Professional's Handbook*. Facet, London.

Huang, X., Lin, J. and Demner-Fushman, D. (2006) Evaluation of PICO as a Knowledge Representation for Clinical Questions. AMIA Annual Symposium Proceedings, pp. 359–363.

Melnyk, B.M. and Fineout-Overholt, E. (2005) *Evidence-Based Practice in Nursing and Health Care. A guide to best practice*. Lippincott Williams and Wilkins, p. 29.

Straus, S.E., Richardson, W.S., Glasziou, P. and Haynes, R.B. (2005) *Evidence-Based Medicine: How to Practice and Teach EBM* (3rd edn). Elsevier, p. 257.

For further resources for this chapter visit the companion website at

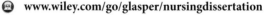 **www.wiley.com/go/glasper/nursingdissertation**

Section 3 **Developing your healthcare/ evidence-based practice dissertation**

Sue and Sam are learning to use the bibliographical databases to kick-start their search for appropriate literature to underpin their dissertations. They have been given access to a complete sample dissertation (which is part of this book's electronic resource) which allows them to see firsthand how the architecture of a dissertation is constructed. Both are conscious of how they must use their time wisely to ensure that they meet the deadlines for writing the various chapters of their dissertations.

Chapter 10   **Managing your time wisely**

Alan Glasper[1] and Colin Rees[2]
[1]*University of Southampton, UK*
[2]*University of Cardiff, UK*

Scenario

Sue and Sam have now got mixed feelings about the task ahead of them. On the one hand they are excited about exploring a topic and learning something new through it. They are also eager to gain their qualification for the work. However, the size of the dissertation is worrying them, as are the demands it will make on their time. Sue keeps thinking of her family and trying to fit things in. Sam is thinking about his job and the other interests he has in life. They both share their concerns and agree it is knowing how to start the work and not let life events take over from the work on the dissertation while at the same time 'having a life!'. Sue has her family, as well as her work, and there are many events that will occur during the time of the dissertation that will be difficult to ignore. Sam also has family obligations and tries to regularly look after his health through sessions at the gym and keep friendship ties going.

Sue and Sam's reactions to the work ahead are very typical of students starting a dissertation. Although this kind of activity often is the last piece of work for a programme of study it is often seen as an almost impossible task because of the work involved; this work will need to be accommodated into an already busy and cramped life. Unless these problems can be seen in context and some action plans developed, the experience of undertaking a dissertation is not going to be a happy one. What is the answer to this problem?

The aim of this section is to consider how to improve time management so that the demands of a dissertation can be integrated with other demands in life. Some key principles will be suggested that will make this easier to achieve.

There are a number of things that must happen at the start of your dissertation period. Firstly, the activity of undertaking a dissertation must be seen as an opportunity and not a threat. Secondly, the activity needs to be

---

How to Write Your Nursing Dissertation, First Edition. Alan Glasper and Colin Rees.
© 2013 John Wiley & Sons, Ltd. Published 2013 by John Wiley & Sons, Ltd.

divided into various stages that can then be allocated a time frame that will make the whole job seem manageable. Thirdly, you need to seize control of your time and activities so that you can pace the work to reach the deadline with the minimum of extra stress in your life. So, we are talking about a frame of mind or attitude needed to tackle a dissertation, and then a plan of action that will match a timetable.

A dissertation as a frame of mind

A dissertation will take over your life; it will certainly take over your living space. You may find yourself waking up thinking about it, and it may delay you getting to sleep. This may seem like a nightmare but it does not have to be. The dissertation is something that shows you can work on your own, applying all the skills you have learnt through your programme of study. Often they focus on a clinical or professional problem and when complete they represent your contribution to the professional body of knowledge. If you see it as a growing friend and accept that it will only be in your life for a relatively short period, until the submission date, then it will become more manageable. Your first task is then to make a friend of your dissertation and welcome it into your life.

The second task is to make a space for it in your life. This means seeing it as something that will require you to give it time and provide it with food and nurture so that it will grow in size and, finally, 'move away from home' – your home – once the work is complete. Northedge (2005) suggests you need to become skilled in creating time in which it can sit, either by stopping or reducing an alternative activity, or gaining more time in the week when it is possible to focus on your dissertation.

Scenario

One of Sam's friends who recently completed a master's dissertation, towards the end of his dissertation regularly set his wake-up alarm on his 'iphone' to give him two extra study hours before going to work several times a week. Although he became temporally fixated, other students not so inclined have been known take a month's holiday on a Greek Island and take their notebook computers and write the dissertation in one hit. Whatever works for you!
   The former is usually safer than the latter.

For many people it may simply be a better use of scheduled time and putting some things on hold for the duration of the dissertation. The example of Sam's friend, however, shows it possible to create time.

To help you schedule your dissertation time, it is useful to divide the whole process into a number of sections composed of a number of activities. This allows you to put a time against each activity and fit it into a space that will allow you to complete it. Together these activities will allow you to complete each section to arrive at the final deadline. If this is to work smoothly, good time management, as Cottrell (2008) observes, is absolutely essential. This is because you must take control of the work, as there will be the minimum of guidance from others. Unlike regular contact modules, there will probably be very few timetabled sessions to help you pace your dissertation work.

The whole dissertation can be seen as a beginning-middle-end. Surprisingly, the place to start is the end. This is where you will conclude your dissertation by answering the aim you decided upon at the very beginning of the journey. Now, put the submission date minus two weeks as the finishing point. This will give you a margin of two weeks to get it bound if you need a hard copy or ready for submission. Then take a further two weeks off for the final editing of the sections and making sure there is consistency in things like the headings you have used, making sure that all tables or other 'inserts' are correctly numbered and the contents page is complete with the right numbers against each element. The abstract and acknowledgements may also need to be completed in this phase. You might find it helpful to use a time chart such as a Gantt chart (Chapter 1).

Before your end section, you will need a 'middle' that will contain the bulk of your dissertation. This is often in the form of a review of the literature where you critically examine all the evidence in the form of articles you have collected. For this section you will need to do three things:

1   Source appropriate literature.
2   Read and extract appropriate points from the literature you have sourced.
3   Write rough drafts of the section having decided what goes where and synthesising the material with your own 'voice' so that it leads to a clear conclusion.

The best advice is not to perform these in sequence as separate activities but to do them at the same time. You find it a great advantage to your growing understanding of the topic and your own dissertation if, when you read through your articles, you write some preliminary thoughts in the form of notes for yourself about what other work they may link to, so that this will make the synthesis of the work easier. You may wish to review the sample dissertation guidelines detailed in Chapter 2 before proceeding further.

Now the beginning: this is where you will develop the rationale and background for your choice of topic once it has been decided. The most important tip at this point is to avoid developing your aim until you are quite sure there is accessible information available to build up your dissertation. It is this beginning section that can be the most difficult up to the point that you decide upon the topic that has the appropriate amount of literature to sustain it. This also needs a start time to it and a cutoff point where you start work on the middle section.

Each of the three broad sections will contain the same themes such that the whole dissertation 'hangs together' and develops right the way from beginning to end and flows back again. This means that the beginning may change slightly over time as themes may emerge or get taken out. Whatever themes are in one section must appear in the other sections, so when working on one section you may be able to add some notes for yourself in your draft of earlier or later sections. Always remember any section should always be seen as 80% complete. You may go back and make changes depending on what you encounter or decide later down the dissertation road.

You should now have in your mind three broad sections that all exist at the same time; you will work across these sections at the same time. Although you will be mainly focusing on one section when you work on your dissertation, you may need to add something, even if only a note to yourself in brackets, at the same time in one of the other sections.

In each section there are activities that have to be complete by the end of the dissertation process, so we can now produce your dissertation timetable. Allocate time to each of these activities, looking carefully at your calendar of events making space for family and other occasions that need to be given time. Construct for yourself and your supervisor your work plan that looks something like Table 10.1 which contains target dates for completion. Start with the 'action' list using the ones in the box as a guide, then slot in the dates starting with the last one and work to the present time. If any of them look a little 'odd' or out of sync, you can then make some readjustments. Make realistic target dates and then share that with your supervisor so they can help you to keep to time.

You should now find that you have cut the dissertation down to size by seeing it as a series of activities that need to be project managed against tasks to be completed within a timetable of dates. These dates should dovetail into a social diary.

Conclusion

In conclusion, there are a number of strategies you can employ in order to achieve the best use of your precious time. Planning is a key aspect of dissertations and coordination of the activities that go to make up each part of the work. Get support from those around you and try to keep to a timetable that is realistic and gives you some balance in life. Try and allocate so many

Table 10.1 Example of a dissertation timetable.

Target date	Action
Deadline 1 (write as dates)	Select topic, check literature is there to support it. Start dissertation diary to record progress and key decisions and 'to-do' list. Write draft rationale/background to the topic. Give dissertation a title in the form of a statement, and an aim that begins, 'the aim of this dissertation is to...'; send to supervisor and arrange meeting to discuss.
Deadline 2	Write plan to follow to search literature including databases, key words, time frame, inclusion and exclusion criteria. Search literature following plan, adjusting plan or search as necessary. Keep track of hits per database and how numbers of possible inclusions are reduced into those finally included in literature. As literature is gathered, quickly read, make notes, decide on section to place it and how it will integrate with other work.
Deadline 3	Write search strategy and draft early section of review. Send to supervisor to check approach.
Deadline 4	Complete search of literature section and first draft of review of literature.
Deadline 5	Complete sections following literature review, e.g. change sections, recommendations.
Deadline 6	Before moving into final sections such as conclusions, read through work to date and ensure you have a clear idea of the shape of the assignment and map out where it is going in final sections.
Deadline 7	Complete first draft of whole of dissertation excluding sections before the introduction. Check conclusion matches aim. Check references.
Deadline 8	Complete sections before introduction, such as abstract, acknowledgements and contents page, and check pages in work correspond with those in contents page. Check all tables and boxes have headings and titles and are listed in contents page following main sections under heading 'Tables/Boxes'.
Deadline 9	Complete two weeks on editing, reading to make sense of everything. Check all headings are in a similar format, all references correct and listed. Check dissertation guidelines and requirements against work completed to ensure nothing missing and everything has been considered. Final preparation for submission, any binding, checking method of electronic submissions.
Deadline 10	Submission date. Deliver the dissertation according to plan. Celebrate!

hours a week to work on the dissertation and set a target of so many words per week or per 10 days. Record this in your dissertation diary and you will be surprised at how quickly the words mount up. Do not leave the writing until the very end as you will put yourself under too much stress and lose a lot of the good ideas you had as you went along. When you set yourself a weekly work schedule for your dissertation work, try and add a little time or an extra session so that if something unexpected happens you can be flexible in the way you cope with it. All of these will contribute to you feeling in control of the work, and will not leave you feeling stressed and exhausted. A dissertation is something that should be enjoyed but you need to give yourself time to achieve that.

Scenario

Following this advice, Sue and Sam feel that many of their anxieties about finding time for the dissertation have reduced. It is a lot of work, but they have found that having a clearer picture of the activities and the need to keep pushing forward with it has made it manageable and achievable. They have also ensured that those around them know they are going to need support but that it is for a set period, after which things can return more to normal.

References

Cottrell, S. (2008) *The Study Skills Handbook* (3rd edn). Palgrave Macmillan, Basingstoke, UK.

Northedge, A. (2005) *The Good Study Guide* (2nd edn). Open University, Milton Keynes, UK.

For further resources for this chapter visit the companion website at
   🖥 **www.wiley.com/go/glasper/nursingdissertation**

Chapter 11 Developing your study skills

Alan Glasper[1] and Colin Rees[2]
[1]*University of Southampton, UK*
[2]*University of Cardiff, UK*

Why do we need to consider study skills in this book? It is because at degree level and as part of your dissertation you will need to be an independent learner. There will be fewer people telling you what to do and less 'contact' time to get direction. The direction and major decisions come from you. This means you cannot leave it until it gradually becomes clear to you what is going on; you have to be in control of your own learning and be proactive. Without this kind of approach, you may suddenly find that the dissertation submission date is almost upon you and all you have are some quick notes you made so long ago that you find it difficult to understand what you originally wrote.

The dissertation is about bringing together a large number of skills at the right time so that there are no hold ups or 'dead time' while you are waiting for things to happen. As far as possible you should try to carry out activities in parallel so that you can coordinate task that need to be completed at the same time.

Scenario

Sam is concerned as he has been out of studying a little while that he has for-gotten all the things that make a course and an activity like a dissertation easy. Sue has found she can tackle certain parts of assignments OK, like the reading, which she quite enjoys, but gets a little unsure about what she is supposed to write. They realise that what they need to do is consider their personal strengths and limitations when it comes to study skills.

The aim of this chapter is to consider some of the study skills that are appro-priate to dissertation work. In reading this you will find you are already doing some of them, but you should find that there will be some new ideas that will

---

How to Write Your Nursing Dissertation, First Edition. Alan Glasper and Colin Rees.
© 2013 John Wiley & Sons, Ltd. Published 2013 by John Wiley & Sons, Ltd.

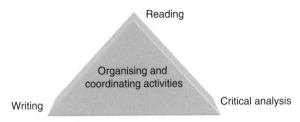

Figure 11.1   Model showing key skills areas in developing your dissertation.

help you get over some of the challenges to dissertation work, especially if you identify with similar issues to Sam and Sue.

The essential skills for dissertations are those shown in Figure 11.1. They are essential as they move the whole activity forward and they must be of the right level to get you the right level mark for your achievements. (NB: you should always aim to get the best classification for your under-graduate or postgraduate degree.) The good thing about them is that they work together, and together make up the key feature of your dissertation. The diagram can be seen as a 'dynamic' model in that each of the corners of the triangle are in constant motion and working with the other parts of the triangle. Wherever you start you must take the other two into account.

One of the key areas in a dissertation is that of critical analysis. This is not an easy idea to convey and a number of sections in this book are designed to help you develop this skill. It does not mean the skill to be critical but to be able to make judgements based on sound principles. At degree level it is showing that you can make balanced judgements and support your comments with reasoning and evidence from other authors to support your statements. This means exploring the statements made by authors as well as considering any assumptions that go with the statements and whether you feel the statements are reasonable and supported by evidence and other authors. Part of critical analysis is indicating to your reader not only what someone says but what you feel about what someone says.

To help you think about developing your skills in critical analysis consider using a simple two-column table (Figure 11.2).

The left-hand column of the table can be used to jot down notes about 'What are they basically saying?' The right-hand column can be used to write down notes about 'What do I think of this, especially the 'so what' of the implications of this?'. Then when reading an article or text book fill in the columns and use this technique until you do not need the columns and you begin to automatically read things with these two questions in mind. This will develop your ability to start thinking critically. Make sure that for the right-hand side you think 'what are the positive things about this, and what are the possible limitations?'; that is, where they are appropriate to the

What are they basically saying?	What do I think of this?

Figure 11.2 Critical analysis skills table.

point. Once you master this skill you can begin to contemplate using the sophisticated critiquing tools discussed in Chapter 19.

Study skills is about how you study by being aware of what time of day suits you best for studying, how long to study at one time before you lose concentration, or if by changing your activity when this happens you can still continue to achieve something in that time slot.

Knowing yourself

Knowing when to seek the help of your friends and supervisor if you start to fall behind your work schedule or if you feel that things are getting on top of you is a valuable skill. These are indicators that you need to do things slightly differently. It is knowing who to approach and being clear in what it is you would like to change. Additionally, if you feel that you may have a learning difference which is impacting on your ability to produce work of a good standard you must approach your faculty learning support advisor as early as possible (see Chapter 27, Managing a learning difference).

Both writing and reading are groups of activities that consist of a number of different elements:

Writing
- Notes for self
- Preliminary 'rough' drafts
- More formal work
- Final draft work

Reading
- Journal articles and recommended text books
- Reading your own notes

The first aspect of managing your reading is finding what to read. Your dissertation will depend on you finding relevant material to answer your dissertation question. One key skill is learning how to make fast and efficient use of databases and not to depend on search engines to do this for you. This is because databases contain work from peer reviewed journals which are a better quality source of knowledge on subjects. To make best use of them check your timetable schedule for programmed sessions on searching databases that might be part of your dissertation module or arrange to attend a session that the university library might organise for students. One of the sections in your review of the literature section will be details on your search strategy and you will need to keep track of the databases you used, the key search words, the time frame covered and any specific inclusion and exclusion criteria that helped you focus down from a large number of 'hits' to a manageable number to include in your literature review. A search details grid may help you keep track of this and some authors have developed search grids for this purpose (Rees, 2010) (Chapter 6, Sourcing best evidence, gives more details of how to use quality databases).

When you find articles you also need to keep track of them, and you may wish to use folders with 'theme' labels to help keep together topic articles that go together.

Extracting information that might be used in your dissertation can also be managed in a grid. The purpose of a grid is to allow you collect information together from different articles under the same column headings, so that you can compare and contrast information from different authors. You will find it an advantage to slot these into a grid so that they appear in year order with the most recent articles first. This has the additional advantage of enabling you to compare trends over time with the findings, sample composition or size, method of data collection and, of course, main findings and recommendations.

You will see examples of these in reviewing the literature articles; they will look like the grid shown in Table 11.2. The headings used here are only suggestions and you can adapt the idea to match the theme headings that are relevant to your dissertation. (A sample of a commonly used grid is detailed in Chapter 15, Introduction to selecting and using appraisal tools/ frameworks: How to interrogate research papers, and this grid is also appended to the companion website www.wiley.com/go/glasper/nursingdissertation.)

For the last column it is always useful to end with 'my comments', in which you include what you found particularly interesting or what may be a possible limitation. This then acts as a prompt for your critical analysis. The grid in Figure 11.3 is presented in 'portrait' format going down the page but you will find it a lot easier to reproduce in 'landscape' format going across the page so the columns are wider and can accommodate more text. Reducing the size of the font size to something like 10 point or even 8 point will also increase how much detail you can include.

Many people find it useful to use highlighter pens to first identify possible information in hard copies of articles before transferring them to a grid. Highlighter pens can also be used to identify the common themes you have divided your review into, so green might highlight problems related to

Author/ Year	Aim	Sample and size	Tool of data collection	Main findings	Recommendations	My comments

Figure 11.3   Example of a data extraction grid.

your topic and yellow possible solutions. Chapter 15 gives details of how to use highlighter pens. These make it easier to pick them out, but also help in telling you at a glance if an article is more 'problem' focused or 'answer' focused. It is techniques like this that will allow you to see the bigger picture and make comments that will get you more marks than just being descriptive.

For reading it is important to become an active reader. This is different from reading a novel where you can just let the words flow over you as the images of the story emerge and take shape. Reading non-fiction is not like that. It is important to remain alive to the messages that a journal article or text book contains. Here it is important to be continually asking questions or 'interrogating the text' in terms of the key messages it contains and the way it fits into what has already been read. One tip is to read the first sentence in each paragraph as that is often the 'topic sentence' that contains the main point of the paragraph. Just scanning down the pages reading the first sentence can often help you to get a total picture very quickly. The same also applies to your drafts, where you can check if your work is flowing by reading the first sentence in every paragraph. There should be some kind of clear narrative when you read first lines. You may need to reconsider how you are presenting material if it does not flow.

Reading each article from your search may take you longer than you think, you can also quickly feel 'saturated' with the information and lose interest in an article, especially if it contains complex terms and statistics. Try not to be too ambitious in each 'reading session' you do. Set yourself to do either just one article or so much of an article, but transfer the information into a grid or make notes as you go along. This will mean you will not have to read the whole article again from the beginning but can read your grid or notes to catch up to where you left off. You will quickly find that the grid builds up and you begin to see the picture it contains based on the articles you have read. Always keep several copies of your papers so that you can have one in your handbag or briefcase which you can read on boats, buses trains and aeroplanes or during your lunch or coffee break

Bringing all the activities together in a coordinated and meaningful way in a space given for your dissertation is important. This is a creative activity and one that you can be proud of the results. It should not be raced through with the aim to get it behind you as quickly as possible.

Being organised

Very few people have too much spare time on their hands, especially when working on a dissertation. The issue is one of prioritising the many tasks you have to complete in the various phases of the dissertation and working out where you should be spending your time so that you make best use of it. Things that might help are 'to-do' lists that are weighted into those that must be done sooner than others. For example, using a coding system of 'A's 'B's and 'C's with 'A's being the ones that must be done before any 'B's and so on. However, it is always worth noting that sometimes choosing some out of this system does provide variety that may influence whether some get done or not.

One important area of prioritising is related to the reading you will have to do. This applies especially when you are reviewing the literature, as there will be a lot to read in a short space of time when you are trying to gain a quick view of articles that will be of help to you. A simple system when you have down-loaded or run-off an article, is to quick scan it, make an assessment of its value and then in the top left-hand corner above the title give it a 1–5 star system rating, with the more potentially useful articles having the greater number of stars. Hence, very relevant up-to-date article may get four or five stars, whilst an older article with only the odd good definition or point will get two or three stars. Sort your articles by star rating and make sure you read the high star articles first. You will be wasting your time if you give equal weight to each article.

A big part of being a successful dissertation student is being very organised with the amount of work you have to cope with. Some of this will relate to clearly seeing how much work you have to do, some of this has to do with making best use of your time. However, some of it has to do with managing the amount of information that you will collect, process and use within the dissertation. Managing files is one area that needs thought. There is also the area of managing your references so that you do not lose material and its original source. You also need to manage references either manually or through specially designed software programmes (Chapter 8) that will keep the details of material you have collected and allow you to reference it in the reference system you are required to use (usually Harvard).

Organising things in terms of what goes where

Try to let your computer to do as much work for you as possible in terms of accessing material, a source for reading on screen and writing directly on screen. Crucially, clearly label files and folders with names that accurately reflect the content. You will have successfully completed academic work in the past. Dissertation writing is the same kind of work but at a different level.

Consolidating your ideas and activities by talking to others about it

Some university departments use action learning sets to encourage students undertaking dissertations to problem solve. It is through meeting and sharing information with others that facilitates the discussion of progress and problem solving activities.

You need to decide where your strengths are at the moment and then decide which areas you need to work on and how you can improve. Certainly talking it over with a friend can help. You can also gain support from a supervisor, although they will expect you to take a certain amount of responsibility yourself for things. The remaining chapters of this book will help you navigate your way through the dissertation journey!

Reference

Rees C (2010) Searching and Retrieving evidence to underpin nursing Practice. In: K. Holland and C. Rees, *Nursing: Evidence-Based Practice Skills*, 143–166. Oxford University Press, Oxford.

For further resources for this chapter visit the companion website at
   www.wiley.com/go/glasper/nursingdissertation

Chapter 12 **Getting the most from your supervisor**

Judith Lathlean
University of Southampton, UK

Scenario

Sam is about to embark on his EBP project and has been allocated a supervisor. Sam knows that the BSc dissertation he did some years ago is quite different from a Master's dissertation. He is keen to get the most out of his supervisor but now he is studying at a different level he is wondering what to expect from the supervisor and is a little overawed at that prospect. Generally, though, he is positive about the chance to work on a one-to-one basis with a knowledgeable member of academic staff.

How to get started

It is best to start on a good footing with your supervisor. Usually a supervisor is allocated to you but sometimes you may have met a lecturer during your programme who seems very interested in your topic idea. If this is the case it is worth asking if they might be able to supervise you, especially if you feel you are on the same wavelength. Otherwise supervisors are allocated according to their knowledge of the subject. Supervision may occur face-to-face, at a distance using multimedia, email or telephone or via group supervision.

You should take the initiative to contact them once you have their details. Do this early – the sooner you can get started the more successful you are likely to be. This shows your supervisor that you are eager to start on your project and keen to get their support. It is also the beginning of a successful relationship and one that will help you to produce the best possible dissertation.

How to Write Your Nursing Dissertation, First Edition. Alan Glasper and Colin Rees.
© 2013 John Wiley & Sons, Ltd. Published 2013 by John Wiley & Sons, Ltd.

Agreeing a working pattern

At the outset you may wish to draw up a research contract with your supervisor and agree a method of contact, including how often you will meet, what you will do when you meet and so on. This will aid the amicable negotiation of mutual expectations at the formative stages of supervision and helps avoid problems later in the supervision process.

As you progress through the year, reflect and set goals with your supervisor for your supervision meetings. Remember that they will not contact you. It is your responsibility and, above all, bear in mind that the chances of gaining a good degree without regular supervision are greatly reduced.

Anticipating and preventing problems

So what gets in the way of a successful EBP project? It is important to be realistic about access to your supervisor. They want you to be successful and work with you, but equally they have other students to look after, usually heavy teaching loads and, if they are active researchers themselves, large research projects to manage. Agree with them how often you will be in contact and put it in your dairy. Then, before you meet, many students find it helpful to prepare a short 'agenda' and after the meeting write a brief note of what you have agreed with your supervisor.

It is vital to maintain a professional attitude to your project, as this will show your supervisor that you are taking it seriously. Indeed the project and dissertation count towards your classification as well as being an excellent way of learning about the research basis of your chosen topic.

It is natural to be anxious about doing well in your project and dissertation, and some students are nervous about revealing their concerns to their supervisor. However, the supervisor will be familiar with this and is there as much to help you with the emotional aspects of working on what may be, for you, an unfamiliar activity, as to provide subject knowledge.

Good planning is the essence

Developing a realistic plan, with manageable timescales, is the key to keeping a project on track. Your supervisor will be able to help you with this, though the project and your ability to complete it is your responsibility. Many students find a Gantt chart helpful (Chapter 1). This lists out the main activities and the time periods. A typical chart is shown in Table 12.1.

The Gantt chart shows when you are seeing your supervisor, when activities will take place, when chapters will be prepared and when the

Table 12.1   Sample Gantt chart.

Tasks	Month 1	Month 3/4/5	Month 6/7/8	Month 9/10	Month 12
See supervisor	▨	▨	▨	▨	▨
Literature searching	▨	▨	▨	▨	▨
Critique papers	▨	▨	▨	▨	▨
Write chapter 1 and 2	▨	▨	▨	▨	▨
See supervisor	▨	▨	▨	▨	▨
Write chapter 3 and 4	▨	▨	▨	▨	▨
See supervisor/write chapter 5	▨	▨	▨	▨	▨
See supervisor with draft dissertation	▨	▨	▨	▨	Finish

supervisor can expect to get some written material sent to them in advance of your discussion.

Preparation of the chart needs you to develop a logical structure for your work. It also implies that you have the knowledge required for the activities, such as the best databases for searching the literature, a critiquing tool such as CASP for handling the literature and an understanding of the methodology if, for example, you are primarily looking at Randomised Controlled Trials. Again, your supervisor may be able to help you, but also there are likely to be sessions in your course that address such aspects or books and articles that you can access to give extra guidance.

Supervision at a distance

Although your supervision may be face-to-face, increasingly students need to make use of other resources too, such as email and Skype. Communication between individuals and groups has been transformed since the inception of electronic means. However, email has to be used wisely. If you have a draft chapter to present to your supervisor for feedback, a good way of conveying it is by email. Nevertheless, do not expect your supervisor to read it and give you feedback by return. A realistic turnaround time should be negotiated with your supervisor at the outset and re-confirmed at various stages during the period of supervision.

Many supervisors are prepared to organise Skype sessions (a type of voice communication service) when meeting in person is not possible. This has the advantage that participants in the session can see each other as well as hear.

Additional support

The supervisor is there to give you support in your project; however, it is expected that you will be able to make the most of this support yourself by being organised and taking the responsibility for your own learning. Many resources are at your disposal – through a whole variety of means. Also, turn to your peers and colleagues; they, too, may have some useful hints, tips and advice.

Activity

Imagine that you are undertaking your own Master's dissertation but you also have experience of your first degree dissertation – an EBP project. Your junior colleague in a neighbouring clinical area – Anna – is doing a top-up programme and over coffee one day you find that her topic is almost identical to the one you did in the past and have subsequently built upon! So you check it out with her and her main supervisor and it is agreed that you will act as more than a peer – rather a co-supervisor for her project.

So what can you expect from Anna and she from you in this role? The answers may be found in the above and you can add to them. In thinking about yourself as a supervisor this should give insight as to how you could relate to your own supervisor.

Box 12.1 Helpful additional suggestions

- In agreeing to be a supervisor you have a responsibility towards Anna. Equally this is her project and not yours!
- If you agree a certain pattern of working with her, try to keep to it unless circumstances change for either of you. In turn you should also expect respect from her; for example, giving you ample warning of problems that are preventing her from progressing or her inability to attend a planned meeting.
- Look for the positives, firstly in her work and then in how she can improve, rather than seeking to critique or criticise her ideas alone. She should expect from you 'balanced' feedback.

Above all – enjoy working with her. The relationship is likely to have some reciprocity. Whilst you will know more than the supervisee, a supervisor can learn something new from every person supervised!

Resources

Critical Appraisal Skills Programme (CASP), http://www.sph.nhs.uk/what-we-do/public-health-workforce/resources/critical-appraisals-skills-programme (accessed 18 May 2012).

For further resources for this chapter visit the companion website at
⓪ **www.wiley.com/go/glasper/nursingdissertation**

Section 4 Preparing to use research evidence in your dissertation

At this point Sam is looking for qualitative studies to use in his dissertation and Sue is looking for Randomised Controlled Trials that will help her answer her dissertation question. One of Sue's friends wants to examine historical literature.

Chapter 13   Understanding quantitative research

Alan Glasper[1] and Colin Rees[2]
[1]*University of Southampton, UK*
[2]*University of Cardiff, UK*

It is not easy to write a dissertation and get good marks without having an understanding of research. This is because research is the major form of convincing evidence you will need to examine and include in your work. However, research can be divided into many different forms; the two major divisions are between quantitative and qualitative research approaches. Your skill in examining an article in a journal will depend on your knowledge of the basic principles of each type. This is because there are major differences in how each type is carried out and how they should be evaluated. Although a subsequent chapter looks at critiquing research, this chapter provides important preliminary information on the way in which quantitative research approaches are conducted. This knowledge will then allow you to evaluate how well studies have followed the principles of this approach.

The primary aim of this chapter is to outline the features of a quantitative research approach and some of the characteristics that make it popular within evidence-based practice.

Is it a quantitative study?

The differences between quantitative and qualitative studies are so different that they are often referred to as two different paradigms, where 'paradigm' means 'world view' (Tappen, 2011). This means the thinking that goes with each type of research approach differs to the extent that they are almost opposites, or at least the sets of ideas about them are quite some way apart. So, for instance, one of the beliefs of the quantitative paradigm is that research is the search for generalisable statements about the constant relationships that exist between variables. Data are seen as objective measurements that can be verified by those with the skills to carry out the measurements.

How to Write Your Nursing Dissertation, First Edition. Alan Glasper and Colin Rees.
© 2013 John Wiley & Sons, Ltd. Published 2013 by John Wiley & Sons, Ltd.

Scenario

At the start of their dissertations, Sue and Sam compared their knowledge on research methods. They both knew that much of the evidence they would spend time reading as part of their literature review would demand a lot of careful consideration where they would have to draw on their research knowledge. Sue's topic of larvae therapy for wound healing in older women with varicose leg ulcers is likely to involve a number of randomised controlled trials (RCTs). She is not looking forward to this as, firstly, she sometimes gets confused between the two terms quantitative and qualitative, and, secondly, because RCTs require a knowledge of statistical terms and principles. Sam also finds the two terms quantitative and qualitative difficult due to his dyslexia, as the words look very similar he does not always notice the difference. As Sam's focus is on the lived experience of families with a child with a chronic illness, his dissertation will mainly draw on qualitative studies, which are covered in the next chapter, but may still contain some quantitative studies to provide some background and clinical detail. They are both looking for some pointers to help them understand how these two research approaches differ and what they may need to take into account when evaluating studies from each area.

Reality is seen as somehow 'out there' and available to researchers through measurement. The qualitative paradigm is different in the way that it feels that 'reality' is inside each of us and we need to construct it through the eyes of those in the setting. In this way there is a different perception on research as an activity and the actions of the researcher within it.

One of the first questions to answer when you locate an article is whether it is a research study. If it is research, it will involve the collection of data from people or things in a systematic way and give clear sections on how the information was collected. There will be a results section that will contain tables or figures, such as bar charts or pie charts, that summarise information collected by the authors and which form the answer to their question or aim. It will not be a review of the literature, which is information collected by other people. It will not be a summary of the research produced by people who have read the original research and it will not be audit, which will relate to findings in one particular clinical setting on the level of service compared to a standard (Gerrish and Lacey, 2010). It will have clear headings, such as aim, method, results, discussion and conclusion, but these will relate to an activity involving the collection of information using a specific data gathering tool.

One of the easiest ways of establishing if it is a quantitative study is to confirm whether it contains tables and figures produced from the results. Usually, you will find this a reasonably successful method of identify research type. This is based on the definition of quantitative research provided by Burns and Grove (2009:22) who defined it as:

'... *a formal, objective, systematic process in which numerical data are used to obtain information about the world. This research method is used to describe variables, examine relationships among variables and determine cause-and-effect interactions between variables.'*

This comprehensive definition highlights that the goal of the quantitative researcher is to turn the data gathered, if it is not already in that form, to a number. So height, temperature, number of children and so on are already in the form of numbers but degree of pain, consciousness or anxiety have to be turned into a number using some kind of scale. This is one of the essential principles of quantitative research.

Why quantitative?

The reason for choosing a quantitative approach is really about the nature of the question the research wants to answer. Topping (2010) agrees, saying the researcher will chose the approach most appropriate for the problem under investigation. If the question requires something to be measured or involves the search for possible relationships between measurable variables, then they will choose a quantitative approach. One of the main purposes of evidence-based practice is to provide the healthcare clinician with the evidence for best practice when there are options available. 'Best practice' is usually seen as an intervention that has the greatest success in improving a measurable clinical outcome, such as a lower level of pain, fewer incidents of readmission or a higher level of physical functioning. A measuring research approach, as provided by quantitative research, is therefore the obvious choice.

Types of quantitative studies

A quantitative approach is a broad term used to describe a number of research designs that produce numerical results. These different include:
- Surveys, which can be descriptive or correlational.
- Experimental approaches, such as randomised controlled trials (RCTs).
- Quasi-experimental approaches, which are similar to RCTs but lack important elements.

The following sections outline some key characteristics of each of these approaches.

Surveys

Descriptive surveys involve a large sample of people, things or events. The purpose of this type of survey is to produce a picture or 'snapshot' in numbers so that the investigators have some ideas of the quantity or size of something, such as the number of people with asthma in a population or the views of patients on different types of treatment options. The aim is to be more precise in the understanding of quantity in regard to events, behaviour and attitudes of a defined group (McKenna *et al.*, 2010). The results are likely to just be an indicator rather than an exact answer, as surveys rarely include the whole population but rather a sample of them.

Surveys can look for patterns of relationships amongst the characteristics they examine by taking a correlation approach. Polit and Beck (2008:272) define correlation as 'a tendency for variation in one variable to be related to variation in another'. For example, is there a pattern that links the social class of people and the extent to which they are following recommended health practices, such as a set level of fresh fruit and vegetables per day, or a pattern between age and type of anaesthesia people would prefer for a certain operation? The purpose of this type of research is more sophisticated and complex than a simple broad descriptive approach, as it allows researchers to predict the number of people who may be more likely to want certain things or be more likely to behave in a certain way. However, the results are again likely to be an indicator and not an exact prediction, as such a pattern may not relate to all people all of the time but will give an idea of a general trend that will be better than no information.

Experimental

Each type of study becomes progressively more sophisticated and complex in its design. One of the most sophisticated types of study is the randomised controlled trial, which comes under the heading of experimental approaches. The emphasis here is often in comparing alternative interventions to see which has the better outcome on a patient's health or recovery.

The experimental process involves a group of people (although it can be objects or events) being randomly allocated to either an experimental or control group. The experimental group receives the variable that the researcher wants to test and the control group commonly has either an alternative intervention, a 'placebo', that is a non-active or 'sham' intervention or procedure, or no intervention. These all allow a comparison between the group with the experimental intervention and what would have happened either without that intervention or in comparison with an alternative.

The important aspect of an experiment is the large degree of control the researcher has in introducing the key 'independent' variable and ensuring that, as far as possible, other variables that make a difference to the outcome or 'dependent variable' are either not present or are present in reasonably equal amounts in both groups through the process of randomisation. For those in an experimental study there should be an equal chance of ending up in either the control or experimental study. Random number generators on computers or good quality electronic calculators are used to allocate subjects in randomised controlled trials.

Quasi-experimental

In some cases where randomising people between two treatment methods is very difficult or raises ethical issues, a less precise form of experiment called a 'quasi-experimental' study is used. Here quasi means 'almost' and looks like a randomised control study with an experimental and control group but does not have people randomly allocated to the two groups; instead it uses groups that already exist, such as people on two different clinical settings who are already part of those settings. So it is almost, but not quite, a randomised control group.

Whereas the analysis of the results using statistical techniques can indicate a 'cause-and-effect' relationship between the variables in an experimental study, in quasi-experimental studies these techniques can only suggest a correlation or pattern between the variables. In this situation the influences of other variables, including the composition of the group, cannot be ruled out. This possibility is reduced through the process of randomisation in a 'true' experimental design involving randomisation. In a quasi-experimental design individuals clearly do not have a fifty-fifty chance of being in the experimental group as they are already in a group before the study begins.

In all quantitative research approaches the emphasis is on accuracy of the measurements used. The tool used to measure the outcomes must be 'reliable', that is, it is consistent and produces stable results whoever is measuring, and repeat measures would produce the same result if repeated immediately. Reliability is an important concept in research and is demonstrated when the researcher uses a tool used in a previous study that is known to measure accurately, for example the Glasgow coma scale or HAD depression scale, or, where no existing tool is available and the researcher designs one that is fit for purpose, a pilot study is used to tests its accuracy or reliability.

Once measurement has taken place, the results have to be processed statistically to see if any relationships exist between the variables using the numbers as a way of indicating this. Statistical tests will indicate the likely existence of a correlation or pattern between variables in a study. Other tests, called 'tests of significance', will establish if it is likely that a cause and effect relationship exist between the variables. A study that can indicate this kind of relationship is the most prized type of research in quantitative research and is often referred to as the 'gold standard', as so much care or control over the process is taken to make the study as accurate as possible. This then permits the results of a study to be generalised, where the results can confidently be applied to other similar situations.

The ability of RCTs to indicate generalisable cause and effect relationships explains their position towards the top of the hierarchy of evidence, which is a way of indicating levels of preference for the type of studies chosen to answer an evidence-based practice question. At the top of the hierarchy of evidence are systematic reviews of RCTs, because of the care taken to produce 'systematic reviews' by only including the most accurate and rigorous research available, which tends to be RCTs. Naturally for dissertation work it is these kinds of studies that would be first the choice, as they allow a student to argue for the use of a particular nursing intervention.

NB: If a systematic review on a certain subject has recently been published it may prohibit the student from actually continuing with the EBP question which they have posed. This is because systematic reviews reassemble the parameters of some dissertation guidelines (but usually much more deeply) and as the whole purpose of completing a dissertation is to learn the skills of searching and critiquing literature, the existence of a recently published systematic review which does just that would undermine this.

Key elements in a quantitative study

When reading a quantitative study there are a number of elements you need to consider that will indicate the quality of the study and its relevance to your dissertation. These are covered further in Chapter 15 on critically appraising evidence, so only preliminary points will be included here.

Having established that it is a research study, and confirmed it is a quantitative design by the presence of numbers either in tables or in the results section, look for the elements identified in Table 13.1. The table uses some of the familiar research terms you will meet in research studies and these are the words that will indicate your understanding of research in your dissertation. Using them will help achieve better marks. Check in the glossary of terms in Chapter 24 if there are any terms that you need to clarify.

Table 13.1 provides you with a guide to the structure of most articles and the elements that you need to locate and consider. They will help you build up a picture of the similarities and differences in studies you have found and enable you to start the critiquing process.

Strengths of quantitative studies

Quantitative studies are seen as the most desirable form of evidence for evidence-based practice. This is because of the many principles followed by quantitative researches, such as the use of accurate measuring tools, which provides objective and visible outcomes similar to other 'scientific'

Table 13.1 Key elements in a quantitative study.

Element	Where found	Why important	Look for
Variable(s)	Title, abstract, introduction, results	Helps confirm it matches key variable(s) in your work	How variables are defined and measured (concept and operational definitions). Compare these to other studies.
Aim	Abstract, just before or after heading 'Method' or similar term	This identifies what the researcher is trying to achieve through collecting data	Will this help the purpose of your dissertation? Compare this to other studies to check if they look at similar questions.
Type of study or research design	Title, abstract, methods section	Within quantitative and qualitative designs, each type has its own 'brand' appearance and follows clear principles	Although some studies will say 'qualitative' few say 'quantitative', but will indicate if it is a survey, experimental, randomised controlled trial (RCT), quasi-experimental, correlation or correlational design. Does it match the aim?
Research method/tool of data collection	Abstract, methods section	Shows how data were collected	Is it appropriate for aim, approach, and sample? How accurate or reliable is it? Was accuracy checked by using a previously used tool or through a pilot? *(Continued)*

Table 13.1 (cont'd)

Element	Where found	Why important	Look for
Sample	Abstract, methods section	Problems of bias or lack of convincing evidence can be related to the size of sample and way they were chosen.	Clear inclusion and exclusion criteria, statement of sampling method. Size of sample should take into account variations in population and allow convincing results. Is sample relevant to aim and your dissertation? Is anyone not covered in criteria that might affect relevance? Is size of sample comparable to other studies and seems sufficient? Is method of choosing sample clearly described? Is size of those 'lost' to the study or not responding to the study a problem?
Ethical approval	Methods section	Studies using patients or staff should be approved by ethics committee or, if American, Institutional Review Board (IRB)	Ethical issues raised by the process of recruiting people, or what is done to them. Check for mention of an ethics committee or IRB if any concerns.
Results	Abstract, results section	Should answer the aim	Are the results convincing or are there any limitations or uncertainties? Does this help answer your dissertation aim?
Tables, figures, text figures	Results section	Will indicate part of answer to aim and statistical test values will indicate any relationships	Story suggested by figures. Good statistical values, e.g. $p < 0.05$, or better, e.g. $p < 0.01$

Element	Where found	Why important	Look for
Main findings	In any tables or figures and text of the results section	Answers the aim of the study	Do the results build up to a clear answer to the aim which provides you with evidence for your dissertation.
Conclusion	Abstract, end of discussion under heading 'Conclusion'	Will answer aim; anything that includes 'should' is a recommendation not a conclusion	Compare with other studies. Positive results to support your dissertation aim.
Recommendations	Abstract and after conclusion	Will suggest 'best practice' and implications for practice	Statements containing 'should' as these indicate a recommendation. Compare these with other studies. Support your 'change' section and 'application to practice' in your dissertation.

disciplines such as physics and chemistry. The method of collecting data in these studies is described in detail so that they can be repeated or reproduced to check for accuracy and rigour. In this way, high quality 'rigorous' studies, that is, ones that show the researcher's ability to produce accurate results, allow us to generalise the conclusion to other settings as care is taken in making the sample as close as possible to the larger group they represent.

Limitations

Despite the strengths noted above, quantitative research also has limitations. For example, not everything that should be taken into account when deciding between alternative interventions is based on measurable outcomes. There are other considerations, such as the quality of care, or the wishes of the individual for the kind of intervention or, indeed, whether they will accept an intervention, that are just as important. In other words, quantitative results are only a part of the picture.

Some studies lack the rigour required to make the results strong enough to consider, often due to too small a sample or aspects of the study that have introduced bias into the results and conclusion.

Conclusion

Quantitative research is a major element in evidence-based practice because of its emphasis on accuracy and transparent methods of data collection. Knowing the structure and principles of the major forms of quantitative research will help you answer dissertation questions that relate to best practice. The 'gold standard' for this kind of approach is the randomised controlled trial, as this demonstrates the greatest degree of control by the researcher. It also is the method that indicates cause and effect relationships that allow clinical options to be chosen with reasonable confidence. Each study should be carefully examined to ensure that it conforms to the methodological principles of this kind of study. Although quantitative approaches have many advantages, there are still aspects that in healthcare need the balance provided by qualitative approaches. This research design forms the subject of the Chapter 14 (Understanding qualitative research).

References

Burns, N. and Grove, S. (2009) *The Practice of Nursing Research: Appraisal, Synthesis, and Generation of Evidence* (6th edn). Saunders, St Louis.

Gerrish, K. and Lacey, A. (eds) (2010) *The Research Process in Nursing* (6th edn). John Wiley &Sons Ltd, Chichester.

McKenna, H., Hasson, F. and Keeney, S. (2010) Surveys. In: K. Gerrish and A. Lacey (eds), *The Research Process in Nursing* (6th edn), 216–226. John Wiley &Sons Ltd, Chichester.

Polit, D. and Beck, C. (2008) *Nursing Research: Generating and Assessing Evidence for Nursing Practice* (8th edn). Lippincott Williams and Wilkins, Philadelphia, PA.

Tappen, R. (2011) *Advanced Nursing Research: From Theory to Practice*. Jones and Bartlett Learning, Sudbury.

Topping, A. (2010) The quantitative-qualitative continuum. In: K. Gerrish and A. Lacey (eds), *The Research Process in Nursing* (6th edn), 129–141. John Wiley & Sons Ltd, Chichester.

For further resources for this chapter visit the companion website at

   📖 **www.wiley.com/go/glasper/nursingdissertation**

Chapter 14   **Understanding qualitative research**

Alan Glasper[1] and Colin Rees[2]
[1]University of Southampton, UK
[2]University of Cardiff, UK

In this chapter we will examine the second major paradigm used in healthcare decision making, that of qualitative research. This is a different way of thinking about research and how a study is conducted compared to that of quantitative research. The choice of which method to use is dictated by the nature of the research question the investigator is trying to answer. It is important that each approach follows a systematic and clear method that is described for the reader to judge the quality of the study outcome.

Scenario

Sam is trying to develop a better understanding of qualitative research methods as his dissertation examines the 'lived experience' of families with a child with a chronic illness. He has chosen this topic as he wants to explore some of the issues that such families face. He knows that the term 'lived experience' is related to a phenomenological qualitative approach to research, but the terminology itself is very scary. He is trying to sort out how qualitative research differs from quantitative and he has read some very dismissive comments about this type of research. He feels that until he has a better understanding it is difficult to carry on with examining qualitative research with confidence. His dyslexia does not help

---

One of the problems with qualitative research is that, as its spelling suggests, it concentrates on 'quality' issues, when it is more accurate to say it looks at experiences, interpretations and understandings as defined by those involved in a study. Whereas quantitative research can look at inanimate

---

How to Write Your Nursing Dissertation, First Edition. Alan Glasper and Colin Rees.
© 2013 John Wiley & Sons, Ltd. Published 2013 by John Wiley & Sons, Ltd.

objects such as types of thermometers, walking aids, mattresses or methods of teaching, qualitative research always involves human beings. Holloway and Wheeler (2010:3) define qualitative research simply as 'a form of social inquiry that focuses on the way people make sense of their experiences and the world in which they live'. This emphasises many of the aspects of qualitative research, such as concentrating on how people themselves define a situation. They are not asked to choose from a number of alternatives, as in a questionnaire constructed from how a researcher interprets the world and what may be important. Qualitative research attempts to see the world through the eyes and interpretations of those in a particular situation.

The data gathered in qualitative research are usually in the form of words and that is how they are presented in a section typically called 'findings' as opposed to 'results', although this convention can sometimes be broken, often in ignorance or because of the conventions of the journal in which it appears. As qualitative research does not 'count' anything or use a measuring tool to statistically examine numeric relationships between variables, there are no tables of figures forming the results, apart from a description of the characteristics of the sample. The whole way of thinking about this type of research is therefore different. This has led to some supporters of a quantitative approach to research methods rejecting the value of qualitative research in sometimes quite dismissive or 'name-calling' ways (Tappen, 2011:35). Again this is often more as a result of a lack of understanding of both the systematic way such research is undertaken and the value it can provide to healthcare decision making.

Why qualitative?

There is a clear compatibility between qualitative approaches to research and nursing. This is brought out by Holloway and Wheeler (2010:11) when they point out that it takes 'a person-centred and holistic perspective', which is the same as healthcare professionals such as nurses' approach to individual care. This approach provides insight into the experiences of patients and clients of health services so that practitioners who have not experienced particular situations can begin to appreciate how it is for those concerned and provide a more sensitive and understanding form of care.

This approach does not replace but rather provides the balance or triangulation to a quantitative research approach. Although it is sometimes criticised for being very subjective and very descriptive, it is carried out in the same rigorous way as quantitative approaches, following clear principles of research and an emphasis on the accuracy of the findings.

Types of qualitative studies

As with quantitative approaches, there are a number of different designs grouped under the heading of qualitative research. Although there are many variations, there are three main types that predominate in nursing:

- Phenomenology
- Ethnography
- Grounded Theory

There is also a fourth 'general' category that can be said to follow the general principles of qualitative approaches but does not follow any one approach in particular.

Phenomenology

This approach has developed from philosophy where there is an emphasis on an individual's 'lived experience' of a situation. Often this kind of study will incorporate 'lived experience' into its title or aim; it is the approach that Sam is looking at in his dissertation. The method of data collection frequently used in this approach is in-depth interviews. They are not a question and answer format like a questionnaire but follow a very general opening such as 'tell me what it is like to be the parent of a child with asthma', and then further questions will depend on what the respondent says. The follow-up questions will usually be requests for more details or illustrations of a point. There can be a loose structure of key topic areas to be covered in an interview but the aim is to produce spontaneous thoughts, interpretations or descriptions with the minimum of prompting from the interviewer. This conforms to the unstructured and flexible nature of qualitative methods (Tappen, 2011), where the intention is to capture rich detailed data in the respondent's own words. These lengthy verbal details produced in interviews are then analysed for common themes that emerge within them.

As with all these qualitative approaches, there are a number of variations within each one and you will find different models or guides being followed. Names such as Hursserl, and Heidegger, who developed the thinking on the philosophy of phenomenology may appear, and Giorgi, Colaizzi or Van Manen may be cited in relation to the methodology, particularly in relation to the analysis of the data.

Ethnography

This type of study involves the observation of groups of individuals who share a common 'culture' to understand their pattern of behaviour. Often referred to as gathering data in 'the field', this type of research developed from anthropologists whose aim was to make sense of and describe the culture of remote tribes. In healthcare this has been used to look at the culture of different patient groups and even staff groups. Data are collected over periods of weeks, months or even years and consist of more than one form of data collection, such as observation, interviews and documentary methods. Researchers frequently keep a 'field diary' where their own thoughts, feelings and interpretations are captured and become part of the analysis and interpretation of the setting and its events.

The key to this kind of research is in the analysis where themes emerge from the rich 'thick' descriptions (Holloway and Wheeler, 2010) using a structured form of analysis which is usually carefully described. In common with all forms of qualitative research this analytical approach takes an 'inductive' approach, where the pieces of data are put together to form a view or interpretation of what it going on in a 'bottom up' sequence.

Grounded Theory

Whereas the last two types of research attempt to *describe* human situations and issues, the grounded theory approach, developed by two sociologists, Glaser and Strauss, attempts to *explain* or develop a theory to fit the situation. This theory is 'grounded' in the data that has been collected. Such studies sometimes express the theory in the form of a diagram that shows how all the ideas in the study fit together. In the same flexible, indicative process as previous approaches, it uses a mix of interviews, observation and documentary sources to construct its findings.

Key elements in a qualitative study

The differences between quantitative and qualitative studies can appear quite stark, as almost every aspect can look different. The two constants are the close attention to ethical rigour, where the same guidelines for the relationships between researcher and those involved in a study are protected, and on the outcome of the study matching the data collected as closely as possible. Both of these can be referred to as the rigour of the researcher in carrying out the study to the highest possible standards to ensure that quality of the results.

The key elements of a qualitative study revolve around the attempt to construct a view of the social world of the participants in a study from their own perspective and by concentrating on the richness and depth of information that is possible from the processes involved.

As can be seen from Table 14.1, which compares the two approaches, each aspect of the research process demonstrates differences. Firstly, the research question is broader and more general. Sample sizes are usually smaller as the emphasis is on the depth of data collected from each person. The sampling method does not try to match the sample to the population

Table 14.1 Comparison between key aspects of quantitative and qualitative research approaches.

Element	Quantitative	Qualitative
Aim	Specific and measurable.	Broad question not answerable numerically.
Purpose	Provide accurate answers to questions often involving the relationship between variables, either in a correlational or cause and effect relationship. Seeks to provide 'an answer' to a clear problem that can be generalised to other situations.	Provide insights, experiences and interpretations. Seeks to provide variations in the way that people experience key health issues. Does not set out to generalise findings but increase understanding.
Ethical considerations	Great emphasis placed on confidentiality, avoiding harm and gaining informed consent. If involving patients particularly on health premises by health professional researchers, must get permission of an ethics committee.	Same emphasis on doing no harm (including psychological or social), and gaining consent. However, as some studies do not involve patients on health premises, permission may not always be gathered from a health service ethics committee
Tool of data collection	Emphasis on accuracy and consistency of measurement to ensure standardisation of the tool.	Often more than one tool used. There is flexibility in the use of the tool. In many respects the researcher almost becomes the tool of data collection through their dealings with people in the setting and recording what they see and hear.
Viewpoint	The researcher's viewpoint drives the study through the power and control they have in the situation.	The respondent's viewpoint is the major perspective used. This can be 'interpreted' through the researcher but they attempt to preserve the respondent's construction of how they see things.
Method of analysis and data presentation	Objectively derived from statistic processes. Results are presented in the form of numbers.	Researcher's interpretation of what they feel the data are saying. Systematic procedures followed in the analysis of the data. Findings are presented in the form of words, often under theme headings.
Sample size and selection	Emphasis on large samples selected using processes that ensure they are closely representative of the total population they represent.	Can be quite small but should have experienced the situation in which the researcher is interested. Selection procedures are less elaborate as generalisability is not an issue.

Table 14.1 *(cont'd)*

Element	Quantitative	Qualitative
Generalisability	Research processes should lead to high levels of generalisability.	The aim is to heighten awareness of some situations but there is no primary emphasis on making them generalisable.
Application to practice	High in relation to the question posed. Highly valued within evidence-based practice.	High in relation to the question posed. Not highly valued in evidence-based practice but useful in issues of quality of care and ensuring a sensitive approach to individuals is achieved.

in the same way as quantitative research. The tool of data collection is far more flexible and does not attempt to be standardised, as it is not accurately measuring something but responding to capturing experiences or interpretations. This means the method of analysis in working with text or observations is very different, although frequently very systematic and follows the processes outlined by key writers of this type of research, such as Giorgi, Colaizzi or Van Manen. There is often the use of more than one tool of data collection to try and capture different aspects of the topic. This results in a certain amount of blending of findings in order to build up a clearer picture of the topic.

The interpretation of the data means that the thinking of the researcher is more an inductive approach building up to the suggestion of a bigger picture or theory rather than the deductive approach of quantitative research, which often attempts to apply a theory or bigger picture to the data to establish support for such a theory.

Strengths of qualitative studies

The major strength of qualitative studies is that they provide a rich and productive insight into human experiences in relation to health and illness issues. This produces a depth of understanding of human experiences (Houser, 2008). This knowledge is quite different from quantitative studies as they are located more in the social world of health and illness rather than a medical model's focus on the body and the fight to regain health through interventions carried out by health professionals. The methods used by researchers are just as systematic as quantitative researchers, although very different in their characteristics, and the methodology sections of research articles should be just as transparent in revealing how the study was undertaken, especially the data analysis.

Limitations

Perhaps one of the greatest limitations of qualitative research is the mistrust amongst some health professionals that the conclusions of this type of research are not to be trusted as the interpretation of the findings are very much those of the researcher involved. Polit and Beck (2008:17) suggest that for some people the concern is whether two different qualitative researches would reach the same conclusions from the same data. There is also the problem of whether findings can be generalised, as they are based on small samples.

The two major methods of interviews and observation popular in qualitative research also raise problems. Firstly, with interviews there is the difficulty of 'self-report' data, where there may be a difference between what people say they do and their beliefs and what they actually do and what their beliefs really are. In observational studies there is the problem of 'observer effect', where the presence of an observer may influence the behaviour of people being observed. An additional problem in observation is the inability of the researcher to 'see' everything and cover events or activities that are taking place simultaneously or in neighbouring locations. A certain amount of selection then is inevitable (Holloway and Wheeler, 2010).

Conclusion

Qualitative methods provide the balance to the more numeric and measurement orientated approach of quantitative research. The aim is to provide insights that allow nursing staff to provide a sensitive and insightful level of support. The holistic approach of the method is in keeping with that of nursing, which emphasises the total situation of the individual within their normal environment and not just the medial aspects of their life. This provides a depth of understanding that goes to the heart of the experience as described by those involved.

It is possible to have studies that combine quantitative and qualitative approaches, in mixed method studies. Here the aim is to provide balance and also to contribute to untangling frequently complex health situations (Simons and Lathlean, 2010). However, the majority of research tends to be from one methodological approach or the other. Evidence-based practice provides the scope to use studies from each paradigm to combine best clinical practice suggested by quantitative approaches with the insight and values of patients, clients, relatives and clinical staff as revealed by qualitative studies.

References

Holloway, I. and Wheeler, S. (2010) *Qualitative Research in Nursing and Healthcare* (3rd edn). John Wiley & Sons Ltd, Chichester.

Houser, J. (2008) *Nursing Reaerch: Reading, Using, and Creating Evidence.* Jones and Bartlett, Sudbury.

Polit, D. and Beck, C. (2008) *Nursing Research: Generating and Assessing Evidence for Nursing Practice* (8th edn). Lippincott Williams and Wilkins, Philadelphia, PA.

Simons, L. and Lathlean, J. (2010) Mixed methods. In: K. Gerrish and A. Lacey (eds), *The Research Process in Nursing* (6th edn), 331–342. John Wiley & Sons Ltd, Chichester.

Tappen, R. (2011) *Advanced Nursing Research: From Theory to Practice.* Jones and Bartlett Learning, Sudbury.

For further resources for this chapter visit the companion website at
www.wiley.com/go/glasper/nursingdissertation

Section 5 **Critically appraising evidence**

Having collected some relevant research articles, both Sue and Sam are faced with selecting an appropriate critical appraisal tool to evaluate their selected papers. Sam has been advised to use Parahoo's critiquing approach.

Chapter 15 Selecting and using appraisal tools: How to interrogate research papers

Alan Glasper[1] and Colin Rees[2]
[1]*University of Southampton, UK*
[2]*University of Cardiff, UK*

Scenario

Sam and Sue have spent time in the library and have conducted a full search of the bibliographical databases. They have also perused the grey literature and have conduced hand searches of archived journals. After applying inclusion criteria and exclusion criteria they have sourced some relevant data-driven research articles and retrieved them. They are both faced with selecting an appropriate critical appraisal tool to evaluate their selected papers. They know that the critical appraisal chapter of the dissertation is the most important aspect of their evidence-based practice dissertations. Now they must make sure they get the best from each article and convey their knowledge using a critical analysis style of writing.

Introduction

This chapter is designed to help students who are writing an evidence-based practice dissertation to fully comprehend the process of critiquing empirical journal papers. In this chapter a range of critiquing models are discussed and, furthermore, in other separate chapters how these models can be used to critique individual papers is described.

How to Write Your Nursing Dissertation, First Edition. Alan Glasper and Colin Rees.
© 2013 John Wiley & Sons, Ltd. Published 2013 by John Wiley & Sons, Ltd.

What is critical appraisal? What are critical appraisal tools? Why is critical appraisal of published research important? What does critical appraisal mean to nurses and other healthcare professionals?

Burls (2009) suggests that critical appraisal is the process of carefully and systematically examining research to judge its trustworthiness, value and relevance in a particular context. Critical appraisal is a process to be learned by healthcare practitioners to enable them to evaluate not only what an article says but also the quality of the research that has produced it. Poor research will not produce reliable results. By following a systematic process, a professional can weigh up its value and relevance for their own area of practice, usually in a clinical domain. Thus, academic critiquing is an essential skill that nurses and others need if they are to use research evidence in contemporary healthcare .These skills facilitate finding and the using appropriate research evidence reliably and efficiently in practice.

Critical appraisal of published research papers is a process that any healthcare professional faced with solving a clinical problem must undertake before attempting to make any change in practice. The method through which healthcare professionals critically evaluate published empirical papers is one which allows the practitioner make a sound evaluation of the worth and provenance of the material reported in specific journals. In identifying the strengths and weaknesses of the published paper, the practitioner can make a value-judgement of the worth of the reported findings and make a decision about its applicability to their own area of practice. The systematic appraisal of papers using a recognised appraisal tool allows the practitioner to make reliable conclusions about the value of the work they are reading and make assessments as to the relevance of the data to their own arena of practice and, importantly, judge if applying the evidence might make a difference to patient outcomes.

If nurses and other healthcare professionals decide and plan to make changes to patient care management they need to be able to:

- Decide if the research being reported has been conducted in such a way to ensure that the finding is both valid and reliable.
- Be able to understand and make sense of the results.
- Decide if the research is strong enough to suggest changes to practice.

There are many different critiquing tools available, some target specific types of study (e.g. qualitative) and some are generic and can be used to appraise any paper. Katrak *et al.* (2004) have shown that there are no tools that are a bespoke fit to healthcare research and that the interpretation nurses make after a critical appraisal of an individual research paper needs to be considered in light of the individual critical appraisal tool which has been used.

What is the best critical appraisal tool to use?

It is beyond the scope of this chapter to discuss the full range of available critiquing tools available. Most of them are very similar and all are intended to help readers more fully understand the various elements of published empirical papers. Some, such as CASP, have been designed specifically for certain types of paper, for example randomised controlled trials. The University of South Australia International Centre for Allied Health Evidence (http://www.unisa.edu.au/cahe/Resources/CAT/default.asp) offers a full and comprehensive discussion of the attributes of many popular health care critiquing tools. Additionally the Scottish Intercollegiate Guidelines Network (SIGN) has developed evidence based clinical practice guidelines for the National Health Service (http://www.sign.ac.uk/methodology/checklists.html).

All healthcare professionals need to develop the skills of critiquing research-based papers. Critical appraisal is the systematic and unbiased detailed examination of all the reported elements of a published paper or study to allow judgement of both the merits or strengths and the weakness or limitations in order to facilitate both the meaning and relevance to practice (Burns and Grove, 2009).

Many professionals when they first encounter the term critique mistakenly think of the verb 'to criticise', but in this context the word has a different meaning. A critique is a constructive evaluation of a piece of published work which is intended to be objective, unbiased and impartial, taking a balanced view of both the content of the paper and of the research process which has been used by the author(s).

Critiquing is a skill that requires practice. Although there are many critiquing tools available, this chapter will consider critiquing tools which have been developed by:

1 Crombie
2 CASP
3 Parahoo
4 Rees

Some critiquing tools have been designed for analysing different types of research approaches. For example, CASP has a whole suite of critiquing tools and Rees has developed a tool for the analysis of both qualitative and quantitative papers, whereas Crombie and Parahoo have developed one model which can be applied to all types of published research. Later chapters in this

> **Box 15.1**   How many papers should be critiqued for an evidence-based practice dissertation?
>
> This will vary from university to university but for some undergraduate dissertations there is an expectation that the student will use a minimum of three where there is a paucity of published papers up to a maximum of five where there is a significant body of knowledge available. This is where the student can develop a long short list of papers before making a final selection of those papers which best fit the PICO/SPICE question posed and meet the full inclusion and exclusion criteria which have been set.
>
> For MSc dissertations in some universities up to 14 papers may be critiqued to ascertain answers to more complex clinical questions and for a PhD a full appraisal of all pertinent literature is expected.

book show in detail how these tools (namely CASP, Parahoo and Rees) can be applied to specific types of research papers (Chapters 16–19).

Commencing your critique

Before making your final selection of papers to critique it is useful to consider McCarthy and O'Sullivan (2008), who suggest that the first priority when considering applying the critiquing process is to consider if an individual paper is worth reading. How can we do this? The following are questions that will help:

- Is from a peer reviewed journal? This will help indicate if the paper is from a reliable source, such as a well-known professional nursing journal. This can be easily verified by going online to the journal WebPages, where full details of how papers are selected for publication should give details of the peer review process
- Consider the title and whether it is relevant to the topic you are exploring. What does it say? Can you trust it? And will it contribute to your practice?

This process will allow you to develop a 'long short list' of suitable papers that you will consider before making your final short list to engage in the full critiquing review process (Box 15.1). The short list of papers should be clearly indicated in a table at the beginning of the critiquing chapter if your dissertation requires this.

Is an individual paper worth adding to the short list? Preparing your initial long short list

When faced with a choice of papers, the task is to narrow the field to whatever number the university prescribes in its student assignment guidelines. In making an informed decision to prepare a long short list selection you will find it helpful to read the description of what the author(s) examined in the paper and answer these questions:

1   How do they justify the need for the study?
2   How did they carry out the study?
3   What did they find?
4   What did they come conclude?
5   Assess if rigour has been applied to the research process, that is, how well was it thought through and what steps were taken to reduce problems of bias, reliability and validity?
6   What is the study's contribution to your professional practice? For example: Does it provide clear evidence for continuing, adapting or challenging practice? Who might benefit from the study, and in what way?

Now make your final short list selection (consider putting this in a table at the beginning of your own critiquing chapter).

Commencing your initial read and review of an empirical journal paper

Before you start and irrespective of the particular critiquing model you have selected for your own dissertation, there are a number of elements that should be considered when critically reviewing a paper. Firstly, reading empirical or data driven research papers is very different from reading a newspaper or a holiday novel. This type of reading is active rather than passive, requiring significant concentration and the burning of many calories by the cognitive centres of the brain! This type of reading requires an active, analytical and reflective approach (Table 15.1). To hone these active reading and analytical skills it is necessary to divide the paper into its constituent parts. Many journal papers are already structured in this way to make their reading more focused. Every journal editor of every health professional journal knows that their readers are busy practitioners with limited time to read. This is why most good journal papers will include a detailed abstract informing the reader of the banner headlines of the study contained within the published paper. Many busy practitioners will only ever get round to reading the abstract but for the purposes of undertaking an evidence-based practice project as part of a university course or as part of professional development it is necessary to drill deeper into the hidden recesses of the paper.

Detailed and methodical reading will help the reader initially gain an outline of the research, and facilitate an understanding of how the various parts of the paper fit together. To become an active reader certain questions need to be asked, which in turn generate answers that help in the decision making process of assessing the relative value of the paper to one's own field

Table 15.1   Stages in critical reading of research articles (LoBiondo-Wood *et al.*, 2002).

Stage	Purpose	Activities or critical questions:
Preliminary understanding (skim or speed read)	Skimming or speed reading to gain understanding of the content and layout of the paper	• Use a highlighter pen to show the main steps in the research process • Make notes (comments and questions) • Note down key variables • Highlight new or unfamiliar terms and significant sentences • Look up unfamiliar terms and write in definitions
Comprehensive understanding	Increasing understanding of concepts and research terms	• Review all unfamiliar terms before second reading • Clarify any additional terms • Read additional sources as necessary • Identify how the main concepts relate to each other and the context of the study • Write brief summary of the main idea or themes of the article in your own words • Identify any further questions or areas that need further clarification
Analysis understanding (breaking into parts)	Break the study into parts; understand each aspect of the study. Relate to steps in the research process At this point you can start to critique the study using a critiquing framework or criteria, applying them to each step in the research process	• What is the purpose of this article? • Am I clear about the specific design used, so I can apply appropriate critiquing criteria? • How are the major parts of the article related to the research process? • How was the study carried out? Can I explain it step by step? • What are the researchers' main conclusions? • Can I say I understand the parts of the article and summarise them in my own words?
Synthesis understanding	Pulling the above steps together to make a (new) whole, making sense of it and explaining relationships	• Review notes on how each step compared with the critiquing criteria • Briefly summarise the study in your own words, identifying the main components, and the overall strengths and weaknesses • This is a critical commentary on the study rather than a description or précis of it

of practice. The various critiquing tools available for practitioners to use provide such a question framework

Points to consider about the paper(s) before using any critiquing tool

1 **Focus**

This is the first aspect to be considered when starting to read a paper, as this allows the reader to put it in the context of existing knowledge about the subject. This is usually stated in the opening paragraph or separately as simply words, concepts or variables covered in the article. Often the title of the paper conveys at least some of this but cannot be relied upon to do so. *Here, you as the reader are making a judgment about the sphere of the paper content.*

2 **Background**

The abstract and opening paragraphs should convey the background to the study and readers should expect to see citable evidence as to why the particular topic is a problem worthy of investigation (e.g. pain relief after spinal surgery or larvae therapy to promote wound healing). Most studies should begin with a definition or an identification of the practice area problem and this will be followed by a broad review of the contemporary literature pertinent to the subject. *Readers should expect the authors to be critical in their own appraisal of the literature being reviewed!* Importantly, use this to identify the strengths and weaknesses of previous studies to illuminate the reasons why the current study has been undertaken and reported. In this section of the paper authors will present the overall framework of the study.

3 **Study aims, hypothesis or objectives**

These should be clearly stated and should emerge after reading the initial part of the paper. Usually the aim/hypothesis or objectives will be cited first in the abstract and then more comprehensively described within the body of the paper.

4 **Methodology**

This section should be simply stated in the abstract, and then in more detail under a heading of method/methodology. This aspect of the paper should identify the research design of the project. The research design should be appropriate to the research questions. Some research questions will require a qualitative approach, for example patients' perceptions of ambulatory day care surgery versus inpatient care. Others may require a quantitative approach, for example the effect of gentle exercise on blood pressure measurement in the elderly. Irrespective of the design, the authors of the paper should give sufficient detail of the methods they have used to elicit data to answer the original research question or topic area they have posed. Authors should acknowledge both strengths and weakness of the data collection tool and give details of any other data collection method they might have used in endeavouring to triangulate their data, that is, look at the topic using more than one data collection tool to ensure the accuracy of the results.

Scenario

What nurses say and do about healthy eating. Using triangulation to support or reject study findings.

Sam has been chatting to Sue about one of his postgraduate colleagues who is a senior health visitor undertaking a taught Doctorate in Clinical Practice. She has used a quantitative survey questionnaire in an attempt to measure life styles of a cohort of student nurses and, in particular, what they eat. Additionally, to help triangulate or corroborate her findings she has interviewed a subgroup of the cohort using a qualitative semi-structured interview schedule. Surprisingly, what she found was that rather than confirm the veracity of the survey instrument findings, the student nurses at interview demonstrated that what they said in the survey and what they actually did was very different. Hence, the sample of nurses revealed, at interview, to drinking more alcohol, smoking more cigarettes and eating more high fat content ready meals than they had admitted to in the survey.

Good papers will also in the method section give detail of any pilot work undertaken as part of the study. This helps to strengthen the validity of the research tools they have used, for example all questionnaires should be piloted.

5 **Ethical considerations**

All reported studies published in journals should acknowledge the ethical issues related to among others, consent in the study. The reader of the paper should be able to ascertain that the researcher(s) have gained ethical approval (Chapter 29 💬).

6 **Main findings**

All published studies should give clear details of the main findings of the research, either qualitative or quantitative. How the results are displayed is also important. It is very important to note that it is not expected that the authors of the papers will define and explain the statistical terms they have used; is assumed that readers will be familiar with the various tests used by the researchers. Practitioners initially find the world of healthcare statistics a mine field of confusing numbers, symbols and words. In Chapter 24 we present a glossary and definition of popular statistical terms.

7 **The discussion section**

Following the results section all journal papers should discuss the issues that have arisen from the findings. Additionally, the researchers should comment on any limitations to the study, for example small sample size or poor response rate to a questionnaire. It is also usual for papers to cite the findings of other similar studies to compare or contrast the findings with their own.

8 **Conclusion**

Published papers should always include a conclusion in which the author(s) briefly sum up their findings and, importantly, the implications, if any, for practice.

Applying a critiquing framework tool of your choice to your selected papers

---

Scenario

Sue has been to the local supermarket where she has bought a large pack of children's highlighter pens, including some exotic fluorescent colours, which she believes will be useful as she now has a different colour for each of the critiquing tool questions. Her idea comes from the work of Riley (1996) who used this as a method of identifying commonalities in transcribed qualitative interviews. Sue has selected four papers to undertake the critiquing exercise. Sam and she joke about the cutting up of the papers colour by colour to facilitate answering the critiquing tool questions across all the selected papers but at least one member of Sam's groups intends to do this. This student also has content lists stuck to the inside of her kitchen cupboard doors! Sue believes that whatever works for the individual is helpful.

Tasks to do before commencing a full critique of a selection of journal papers

Having made your final choice of papers and, before you begin the task of critiquing, it is important to first:

1 Buy a large pack of colour highlighter pens. These can be obtained in most supermarkets and are invaluable in the critiquing process.

2 Have at least three or four copies of each your selected papers: one to carry with you in your handbag, briefcase or rucksack to read on the bus,

Author (Year) Country	Aim(s) of study	Methodological Issues		Relevant/ key findings
		Sample	**Design, data collection and analysis, rigour/ reliability and validity**	

Figure 15.1 Savage and Callery Grid.

train or plane or in your coffee break; one to identify specific details using the colour highlighter pens. (Some students like to cut up one copy of the papers with scissors after highlighting and reassemble piece by piece to match the criteria of the specific critiquing tool they are using.) Finally, keep a spare copy for insurance – just in case!

Using Savage and Callery grids to undertake a preliminary critique

Savage and Callery (2000) used specially designed grids (Figure 15.1) to highlight the primary attributes of the papers they critiqued in their literature review of parental participation in the care of their children in hospital. Some students who are writing evidence-based dissertations find this process helpful as a first stage in their critique of the papers they have selected following their search of the literature. After completion, some students find it particularly helpful to print these grids in landscape and on oversize paper (A2), which they then stick on a wall next to their computers. This helps them to see the primary features of all the papers they have selected for critiquing.

Activity

Source the chapter below from the Glasper and Ireland textbook (most academic libraries will have a copy).

Savage, E. and Callery, P. (2000) Parental Participation in the care of hospitalised children: a review of the research evidence. In: E.A. Glapser and L. Ireland (eds) *Evidence-based child health care challenges for practice*, 67–89. Macmillan

Discuss in your learning group how Savage and Callery used a grid to display the primary attributes of the research literature on parental participation.

Remember, before wring your critiquing chapter you should have a short introduction informing the reader which papers you are critiquing as well as an outline of the critiquing framework you have selected.

Critiquing models

The Crombie model of critiquing

Crombie's (1996) concise guide to critical appraisal has been published by the British Medical Journal and is a very useful model to use in understanding the process of critical appraisal of health research. Many practitioners, such as nurses, find it helpful to follow Crombie's framework to help them think about the process of critiquing a research paper (qualitative or quantitative).

1 Why was it done? (Objectives)
   - What was the rationale for undertaking this study?
   - What was the purpose of the study?
   - Was the research question clearly stated?
2 How was it done? (Methods)
   - Was the research design appropriate to address the research question?
   - How was the sample selected?
   - How were the data collected?
   - How were the data analysed?
   - Were ethical issues discussed?
3 What has it found? (Results)
   - Are the findings clearly presented?
   - Do the findings answer the research question?
4 What are the implications? (Conclusions)
   - Were the findings discussed?
   - Are implications for future practice summarised?

The CASP models of critiquing

The Critical Appraisal Skills Programme (CASP) has been designed by Solutions For Public Health (http://www.sph.nhs.uk/what-we-do/public-health-workforce/resources/critical-appraisals-skills-programme) and provides seven different critiquing tools, each designed for different types of study and these are freely available to download from the website. Given the complexity of this suite of tools only two exemplars will be discussed here:

1 Making sense of randomised controlled trials.
2 Making sense of qualitative research.

Each of these tools has been used within this book to critique papers (Chapter 17 uses tool (1) to dissect a randomised controlled trial paper and Chapter 16 uses tool (2) to dissect a qualitative paper).

10 questions to help you make sense of randomised controlled trials
Although this CASP tool poses 10 questions, each question is further subdivided and the full tool with all the subquestions is available through the website to this book at www.wiley.com/go/glasper/nursingdissertation.

1 Did the study ask a clearly focused question?
2 Was this a randomised controlled trial? and was it appropriately so? (Is it worth continuing to read the paper?)
3 Were the participants appropriately allocated to intervention and control groups?
4 Were participants, staff and study personnel 'blind' to participants' study group?
5 Were all participants who entered the trial accounted for at its conclusion?
6 Were the participants in all groups followed up and data collected in the same way?
7 Did the study have enough participants to minimise the play of chance?
8 How are the results presented and what is the main result?
9 How precise are the results?
10 Were all the important outcomes considered so the results can be applied?

These questions are further subdivided and a full example of a critique of a paper using this model can be found in Chapter 17.

10 questions to help you make sense of qualitative research
Although this CASP tool designed to critique qualitative research papers poses 10 questions, each question is further subdivided and the full tool with all the subquestions is available through the website to this book at www.wiley.com/go/glasper/nursingdissertation.

1 Was there a clear statement of the aims of the research?
2 Is a qualitative methodology appropriate? (Is it worth continuing?)
3 Was the research design appropriate to address the aims of the research?
4 Was the recruitment strategy appropriate to the aims of the research?
5 Were data collected in a way that addressed the research issue?
6 Has the relationship between researcher and participants been adequately considered?

7   Have ethical issues been taken into consideration?
8   Was the data analysis sufficiently rigorous?
9   Is there a clear statement of findings?
10   How valuable is the research?

The Parahoo model of critiquing

Parahoo (1997) suggests asking the questions identified in the following sections when undertaking a critique of any research paper, qualitative or quantitative. These questions are further subdivided and a full example of a critique of a paper using this model can be found in Chapter 18.

The Parahoo framework consists of the following headings that are based on the structure most often used to report quantitative studies in research journals, although this model can be applied to qualitative studies. (An electronic copy of this model can also be downloaded from the companion website to this book at www.wiley.com/go/glasper/nursingdissertation.) The headings are:

- Title of study
- Abstract
- Literature review/Background
- Methodology or Design
- Results
- Discussion and interpretation (including limitations)
- Recommendations.

Title of study

Does the title convey the study clearly and accurately?

Abstract

Does the abstract give a short and concise summary of the following aspects of the study?

- Background
- Aim
- Designs
- Results
- Conclusions.

Literature review/Background

- Is the importance of study justified?
- What is the context of this study?
- Does the literature review show the gap/s in knowledge which this study seeks to fill?

Aims/objectives/research questions/hypotheses
- Are the aims of the study clear?

Design of study
- What is the design of the study? Is it the most appropriate for the aims of the study?
- Are the main concepts (to be measured) defined?
- What are the methods of data collection? Are they constructed for the purpose of the current study or do the researchers use existing ones?
- Who collected data? Can this introduce bias in the study?
- In studies where there are more than one group, is there a description of what intervention/treatment each group receives?
- Is the setting/s where the study is carried out adequately described?
- Who was selected? From what population were they selected? What was the precise method of selection and allocation? Was there a sample size calculation?
- Was ethical approval obtained? Are there any other ethical implications?

Data analysis
- Was there a separate section in the paper that explained the planned analyses prior to the presentation of the results?
- Which statistical methods were relied on?
- Is it clear how the statistical tests were applied to the data and groups?

Results
- Are the results clearly presented?
- Are the results for all the aims presented?
- Are the results fully presented?

Discussion
- Is it a balanced discussion? Have all possible explanations for the results been given?
- Are the results discussed in the context of previous studies?
- Are the results fully discussed?
- Are the limitations of the study discussed?
- Are the results discussed in the context of previous studies?
- Are the results fully discussed?
- Are the limitations of the study discussed?

Conclusions/Recommendations
- Are the conclusions justified?
- Are there recommendations for policy, practice or further research?

- Are the results/conclusions helpful for my practice?
- Are the results generalisable?

Funding
- Is there potential conflict of interest (if information on funding is provided)?

The Rees (2011) model for critiquing quantitative research

An example of a critique using the Rees model for a quantitative study can be found in Chapter 19. (An electronic copy of this model can also be downloaded from the companion website to this book at www.wiley.com/go/ glasper/nursingdissertation.)

1 **Focus**

In broad terms, what is the theme of the article? What are the key words you would file this under? Is the title a clue to the focus? How important is this for the profession/practice?

2 **Background**

What argument or evidence does the researcher provide to suggest this topic is worthwhile exploring? Is there a review of previous literature on the subject, or reference to government or professional reports that illustrate its importance? Are gaps in the literature or inadequacies with previous methods highlighted? Are local problems or changes that justify the study presented? Is there a trigger that answers the question 'why did they do it then?'. Is there a theoretical or conceptual framework that helps us to see how all the elements in the study may be related?

3 **Aim**

What is the aim of the research? This will usually start with the word 'to', for example the aim of this research was '**to examine/determine/compare/establish/etc**.' If relevant, is there a hypothesis? If there is, what are the dependent and independent variables? Are there concept and operational definitions for the key concepts?

4 **Study design**

What is the broad research approach? Is it quantitative or qualitative? Is the design experimental, descriptive or correlation? Is the study design appropriate to the terms of reference?

5 **Data collection method**

Which tool of data collection has been used? Has a single method been used or triangulation? Has the author addressed the issues of reliability and validity? Has a pilot study been conducted or tool used from previous studies? Have any limitations of the tool been recognised?

6 **Ethical considerations**

Were the issues of informed consent and confidentiality, addressed? Was any harm or discomfort to individuals balanced against any benefits? Did an ethics committee approve the study?

7 **Sample**

Who or what makes up the sample? Are there clear inclusion and exclusion criteria? What method of sampling was used? Are those in the sample typical and representative of the larger group, or are there any obvious elements of bias? On how many people/things/events are the results based?

8 *Data presentation*

In what form are the results presented: tables, bar graphs, pie charts, raw figures or percentages? Does the author explain and comment on these? Has the author used correlation to establish whether certain variables are associated with each other? Have tests of significance been used to establish to what extent any differences between groups/variables could have happened by chance? Can you make sense of the way the results have been presented or could the author have provided more explanation?

9 **Main findings**

Which are the most important results that relate to the aim? (Think of this as putting the results in priority order; which is the most important result followed by the next most important result and so on. There may only be a small number of these.)

10 **Conclusion and recommendations**

Using the author's own words, what is the answer to the aim?
If relevant, is the hypothesis accepted or rejected? Are the conclusions based on, and supported by, the results? What recommendations are made for practice? Are these relevant, specific and feasible?

11 **Readability**

How readable is it? Is it written in a clear, interesting style or is it heavy going? Does it assume a lot of technical knowledge about the subject and/or research procedures (i.e. is there much unexplained jargon)?

12 **Practice implications**

Once you have read it, what is the answer to the question 'so what?' Was it worth doing and publishing? How could it be related to practice? Who might find it relevant and in what way? What questions does it raise for practice and further study?

Rees (2011) model for critiquing qualitative research

1 **Focus**

What is the key issue, concept or problem the work examines? What are the key words you would file this article under? Are there clues to the focus in title? How important is this for practice and the profession? Is the type of qualitative design included in the title?

2 **Background**

What argument or evidence does the researcher provide for exploring this issue, concept or problem? Is there a review of previous literature on the subject or reference to government or professional reports that illustrate its importance? Are gaps in the literature or inadequacies with previous methods highlighted? Does the literature review examine the concepts or issues that form the focus? Is there an attempt to justify the study within the context of a qualitative research design? If this is grounded theory there may not be a comprehensive review of the literature at this point, although some reference to previous work may be included as an illustration of its importance. There should be some argument or background information to justify looking at this particular subject.

3 **Aim**

What is the stated aim of the research? This will usually start with the word 'to'. There will not be a hypothesis or the identification of dependent and independent variables, as qualitative research answers a level 1 question. There may be an attempt to provide a concept definition for the concept that forms the focus of the study. On the whole you will find the aim very broad and general and not as detailed as quantitative research.

4 **Study design**

There may be an acknowledgement that the study is qualitative in design and then the type of method specified. The main alternatives are: (i) *phenomenological*, which explores what it is like to have a certain experience, such as a delivery, a pregnancy or threatened miscarriage, and how people interpret that experience; (ii) *ethnographic*, where the researcher enters and participates in the world of the subject by listening, observing and asking questions in order to understand their view of the world; or (iii) *grounded theory*, which will identify concepts which arise from the analysis of the data collected and may also suggest a theory or hypothesis that explains or predicts some of the behaviour that has emerged in the study. It is important that the philosophy behind the method suits the intentions of the research.

5 **Tool of data collection**

Here we are interested not only in the technique used to collect the information but also in the amount of detail we have on the circumstances under which the data were collected. This contributes to the credibility of the study. This should include details of the environment in which the data were collected, over what period of time data collection took place, and any other details that allow us to visualise the conduct of data collection. Did the researcher spend sufficient time, either in observing the life and behaviour of the subjects, or in interviewing subjects, to produce sufficient depth to the data? Because of the flexible way that data are gathered and the way the method will change during data collection, a pilot study will not usually be employed. The researcher should, however, include detail of how they have attempted to achieve procedural rigour in the way the study was conducted. Did they check with those in the study that the information collected was accurate (member's check)?

6 **Ethical considerations**

As with qualitative studies, it is important that the researcher has protected the participant from harm and has gained informed consent from those taking part in the study. It should not be possible to identify individuals or places where the study took place where this might affect anonymity. The researcher should illustrate ethical rigour, including, where appropriate, approaching a Local Research Ethics Committee (LREC), or in American studies an Institutional Review Board (IRB), to approve the research.

7 **Sample**

Who forms the sample and what are their basic characteristics? The sample size may be quite small, even down to three or four, but more usually about 10–15. This may be dictated by theoretical saturation, that is, data collection stops once no new themes or categories emerge from the analysis. In qualitative research it is important to assess whether the participants possess the relevant knowledge or carry out the activity in which the researcher is interested. Has the researcher demonstrated that the participants are able to provide relevant information and are not open to any kind of bias? The reader must consider to what extent the findings, theory or conceptual categories may apply to other settings. This contributes to its *fittingness* to be applied elsewhere.

8 **Data presentation**

The data will be presented in the form of description, dialogue or comments from participants. Is this '*thick*' and '*rich*' description? Is there sufficient detail for us to almost feel that we are there? Do the quotes from participants clearly illustrate the concepts they are being used to illustrate? Is there over-dependence on comments from a small number of the participants in the sample? Has the researcher detailed how they ensured that the data were accurately recorded and representative of the data gathered? Is there anything about the circumstances in which the data were collected that could have threatened the accuracy of the data? Is it possible to discover the '*decision trail*' used by the researcher to determine how the raw data was processed into the categories presented in the results section? This contributes to its *auditability*. Given the same data it should be possible, following the decision trail, to arrive at similar categories and conclusions. Does the researcher present the findings in the participant's own words rather than reinterpreting what was said or done?

9 **Main findings**

What are the key concepts or categories developed from the data? Do the concepts and categories presented cover all the data gathered? Were the findings checked either by the participants (members check) or examined by other experts in the field (*peer review*)? Are the main findings credible, that is, have attempts been made to support the accuracy of the results through rigour in the way in which the study was conducted? Does the researcher discuss the findings and relate these to the literature, or do they leave the quotes to speak for themselves?

10 **Conclusion**

Is there a clear answer to the aim? Does the researcher propose a relationship between the concepts and categories developed in the analysis to form a clear conceptual or theoretical framework? Does the conceptual or theoretical framework reflect the data? Has the conclusion been arrived at inductively (built up from the findings)?

11 **Readability**

Does the researcher present the description of the social circumstances described in the research in sufficient detail that one can almost imagine being there, and hear the participants talking and carrying out the activities described? Is it possible to recognise the concepts described as related to practical experience? Is the report written in a simple and understandable way? Is there a clear 'story line' emerging from the research?

12 **Relevance to practice**

Are the findings relevant to practice or professional knowledge? Is it an important area related to current concerns and issues within the profession? Does the research satisfy the criteria of *transferability*, that is, can the findings in the form of the theory, concepts or categories developed through the study be applied to other situations, or are they only applicable to the place and the people where the study took place? Do you feel the research has sensitised you to issues or provided further insight? Has it confirmed views you might have already held?

Scenario

Sam's supervisor has advised him to use Parahoo's critiquing approach, whereas Sue has been advised to use Rees' model. Both students are aware that all the critiquing tools, at some point in the exercise, ask for a consideration of the results section of the papers. Depending on the level of the course, that is, undergraduate or postgraduate, the amount of information concerning statistical information will vary but, for all dissertations, at least a preliminary understanding of the tests used by the researchers is mandatory.

Conclusion

This chapter has endeavoured to give an overview of the process of critiquing research papers and has sought to outline a number of critiquing models used in the appraisal of contemporary healthcare literature. NB: in Chapter 26, available at www.wiley.com/go/glasper/nursingdissertation, Carpenter gives details of how historical literature can be appraised.

Scenario

Sue and Sam have completed their critiquing chapter of their dissertations. They are now in the final aspects of their dissertations and are planning to write a short chapter summing up the relative strengths and weaknesses of the papers they have read and comprehensively critiqued. They have both been advised to include within this chapter a table showing what these are (Figure 15.2).

Study	Strengths	Limitations
1		
2		
3		
4		

Figure 15.2 Strengths and limitations resulting from the critiquing process (Example of blank table for your use. A copy of this can also be downloaded from the companion website at www.wiley.com/go/glasper/nursingdissertation).

References

Burls, A. (2009) What is critical appraisal? www.whatisseries.co.uk (accessed 26 May 2012).

Burns, N. and Grove, S. (2009) *The Practice of Nursing Research: Appraisal, Synthesis, and Generation of Evidence* (6th edn). Saunders, St Louis.

Crombie, I. (1996) *The pocket guide to critical appraisal.* BMJ, London.

Katrak, P., Bialocerkowski, A.E., Massy-Westropp, S., Kumar, V.S. andGrimmer, K.A. (2004) A systematic review of the content of critical appraisal tools. *BMC Medical Research Methodology.* **4** (22) (http//www.biomedcentral/1471/4/22).

LoBiondo-Wood, G., Haber, J. and Krainovich-Miller, B. (2002) Critical Reading Strategies: Overview of the Research Process. In: LoBiondo-Wood, G. and Haber, J. (eds), *Nursing research: Methods, critical appraisal, and utilization.* (5th edn), Chapter 2. Mosby, St Louis.

McCarthy, G. and O'Sullivan, D. (2008) Evaluating the literature. In: Watson, R., McKenna, H., Cowman, S., and Keady, J. (eds) *Nursing Research: Designs and Methods*, 113–123. Churchill Livingstone, Edinburgh.

Parahoo, K. (1997) *Nursing research, principles, process and issues.* Macmillan, Basingstoke, UK.

Rees, C. (2011) *Introduction to Research for Midwives* (3rd edn). Churchill Livingstone, Edinburgh.

Riley, J. (1996) *Getting the most form your data .A handbook of practical ideas on how to analyse qualitative data.* Technical and Educational Services Ltd.

Savage, E. and Callery, P. (2000) Parental Participation in the care of hospitalised children: a review of the research evidence. In: A.E. Glapser and L. Ireland (eds) *Evidence-based child health care challenges for practice*, 67–89. Macmillan.

For further resources for this chapter visit the companion website at

⚪ **www.wiley.com/go/glasper/nursingdissertation**

Chapter 16 Critically reviewing qualitative papers using a CASP critiquing tool

Di Carpenter
University of Southampton, UK

Scenario

Sue, the top-up degree student, and Sam, the MSc student, have identified a range of qualitative papers that they need to critically appraise to assess the strength of the evidence to determine whether a change in practice is warranted. They have both been advised by their supervisor to use 'The Critical Appraisal Skills Programme (CASP) appraisal tool suite. Sam is considering using the version for qualitative research'. CASP has developed several appraisal tools for different kinds of research.

The tool designed to make sense of qualitative evidence has been developed for those who are not very confident or familiar with qualitative research and, as such, provides a starting point. The appraisal tool is copyright protected but it may be used by individuals so long as it is appropriately referenced – the complete tool can be found at: http://www.sph.nhs.uk/sph-files/Qualitative%20Appraisal%20Tool.pdf (Public Health Resource Unit, 2006) and more details about CASP can be found at: http://www.sph.nhs.uk/what-we-do/public-health-workforce/resources/critical-appraisals-skills-programme (NHS, 2012) Sue and Sam are attending a seminar and have been given a piece of qualitative research in order to practice their appraisal skills. The article's title is 'Sick children's perceptions of clown doctor humour' and was written by Katy Weaver, Gill Prudhoe, Cath Battrick and Edward Alan Glasper (2007). They both dutifully read it through first and then read it again more thoroughly to answer the questions posed by the appraisal tool.

How to Write Your Nursing Dissertation, First Edition. Alan Glasper and Colin Rees.
© 2013 John Wiley & Sons, Ltd. Published 2013 by John Wiley & Sons, Ltd.

> **Activity**
>
> Go to http://www.internurse.com/ and source and print a copy of Weaver, K., Prudhoe, G., Battrick, C. and Glasper, E.A. (2007), Sick children's perceptions of clown doctor humour. *British Journal of Nursing*, **1** (8), 359–365.
>
> Most universities subscribe to Internurse and students can access papers free of charge.
>
> Go to the CASP website and download and print a copy of the qualitative tool.

Screening questions

CASP tools always begin with two screening questions which, if they can be answered quickly with a 'Yes', suggest it is worth continuing with the full appraisal process. This is very helpful, as much time can be wasted on doing a full appraisal only to conclude that the article was not very rigorously written and little confidence may be had in its findings. If clinicians are thinking of changing their practice based upon new evidence, they need to know that the research was sound. Greenhalgh (2010:6) warns of the dangers of clinical decision making by 'press cutting' and describes her experiences as a newly qualified doctor of keeping a file of papers from medical weeklies about new suggestions for clinical practice. She discusses how she would often change her practice based on what appeared to be the newest evidence but came to realise that she did not always know whether the studies to which the articles referred had been conducted properly.

With this is mind Sue and Sam set about their task by looking at the screening questions. Sue looked at the first question, which asks whether there was a clear statement about the aims of the research. The CASP tool gives some hints to help answer this question: what was the research trying to discover, why was it important and to what extent was it relevant? Sue looked over the first few sentences of the clown article and thought she could see what it was aiming at. She then looked more closely at the abstract and found that the beginning of the second paragraph clearly stated that the focus of the study was 'the perceived effects of clown humour as experienced by children in a large children's inpatient facility in the South of England'. The main text gave her more specific details, that is, the study was part of a larger piece of work to investigate the impact of clown humour on children and their families and carers. It also provided some insights into why this study might be important and relevant. The authors had claimed that, firstly, there had been few studies to ascertain the therapeutic effects of using 'clown doctors' to relieve sick children's anxieties and, secondly, that there was little evidence to warrant the use of clown humour. She concluded she could answer 'Yes' to the first screening question.

The second screening question asks whether a qualitative methodology was appropriate. Greenhalgh's chapter on 'papers that go beyond numbers' (2010:163–176) gives a succinct overview about the relative merits of qualitative research and suggests that qualitative researchers 'seek a deeper truth' than that produced by exclusively quantitative research, which is interested in 'counting and measuring' perspectives. Qualitative researchers aim to study their participants in their natural setting (rather than in a contrived experimental situation) and are concerned with making sense of phenomena in terms of the meanings people attribute to them. They are keen to understand the complexities of human behaviour (Greenhalgh, 2010:163). Sam thought about this and noticed that the second paragraph of the article stated that crucial to the study 'was the idea of specifically seeking the views of the children themselves, on the benefits or otherwise of clown doctor humour' (p. 359). The study, then, was about children's experiences and data were collected from four wards (the children's 'natural' setting). Sam also concluded he could give an affirmative answer to the second screening question. Having shared their findings thus far they concluded that the article had passed the screening process and they could progress to the eight detailed questions which followed.

The CASP qualitative questions

The first of these continued naturally from the question that Sam had considered so he agreed to answer it. It asked whether the study design was appropriate to address the aims of the research. The CASP tool suggests approaching this question by ascertaining whether the authors justified their research design. Did they, for instance, discuss how they chose their research method? Sam noted they had described the choice of 'draw and write/draw and tell' methods, which they stated were two complementary qualitative research designs. They gave a full account of the relative merits and criticisms of the approach with children although they did not suggest any possible alternative study designs. The rationale for the choice of approach, however, Sam thought, had been given due and comprehensive consideration and was presented in a fair and non-biased way. Sam thus concluded that the research design was appropriate to address the aims of the research.

Meanwhile Sue was contemplating Question 4 of the CASP tool; this was the first of two questions addressing sampling – she had agreed to consider both. Question 4 focussed on the recruitment strategy and whether it was appropriate to the aims of the research. To answer this question fully,

Sue needed to discover whether the researchers had explained why the participants were selected and whether their recruitment had the potential to generate the type of knowledge sought by the study. The particular study the article referred to, although part of a larger research project which included experiences of parents and carers, was concerned with the child-patients' experiences of clown humour and whether it reduced their anxieties. Children were selected between the ages of four and eleven years, as this age group is suitable to engage with the research methods of 'draw and write/draw and tell'. Allowances were made for difficulties with writing and spelling. Eleven years was chosen as an upper age limit as it was thought that senior school children may have been exposed to more negative and 'horror' associations with clowns. The article also discussed the problems associated with recruitment. The researchers had approached forty-two children but initially sixteen did not consent to participate and a further six were unable to complete the second part of the data collection (they were discharged home early or felt too unwell). It was stated in the article that the data collection had been extended by a month to achieve just twenty participants. It was not clear to Sue, however, why twenty children was the chosen number, although she guessed that this was all that were available to the team in the time frame allocated for the study. She had understood that in qualitative research participants were recruited until data saturation had been achieved. Sue did remind herself, however, that even though the article might not have given a complete account of why the number of participants had been selected, the authors were probably constrained by word limit. It was quite likely that the research itself gave due rationale. Had Sue been using the article for her dissertation then she would have contacted the researchers and asked them (contact details were provided in the article).

The fifth question, also concerned with sampling, included eight subsections. The overarching question addressing all of these subsections was whether the data were collected in a way that addressed the research issue. She had firstly to consider whether the setting for the data collection had been justified. Children had been selected from two medical and two surgical wards from a children's inpatient facility in the South of England. Further details were not to be gained from the article and Sue could not tell whether there were only four wards in this inpatient unit. She did not, therefore, think that the setting for the data had been entirely justified within the article. It was very clear, however, how the data were collected. This was the subject of the second subsection and Sue felt confident that the article had given a full description of how the 'draw and write/draw and tell' methods had been implemented and that data were collected about children's feelings on coming into hospital and, subsequently, following a visit from clown doctors. The third subsection was concerned with justification of the methods chosen but this had already been addressed by Sam in question three. This puzzled Sue a little, but she concluded that the 'draw and write/draw and tell' approach was both a research design and a data collection method in a similar way to a survey. Sue thought the distinction between research design and data collection method in the article could have been a little clearer for the benefit of 'novice critiquers'. The fourth subsection asked whether the data collection methods were made explicit. Sue considered this had been demonstrated well in the article and illustrations had been provided for clarification. The fifth and sixth subsections addressed any modifications to the data collection methods during the study and whether the form of the data was clear. She could easily answer 'no' to the first and 'yes' to the second. The final area of 'sampling' for consideration was data saturation. This question had already been triggered for Sue under Question 4, so she felt she had already addressed this, although she stated here that there was no discussion in the article that data saturation had been achieved with twenty participants.

Reflexivity is the focus of Questions 6 and 7 of the appraisal tool. Sam had offered to consider this section and started with Question 6 to determine whether the relationship between the researcher(s) and participants had been adequately considered. The principle data collector was a play therapist based at the hospital in which the study was conducted. The article made no reference to her having made a critical examination of her role, potential bias or influence, despite brief discussion in the methodology section of the difficulty for qualitative researchers not to impose their own views on the children who are the focus of the research. The article did make reference to the fact that the clown doctors were cognisant and supportive of the study, had no previous knowledge of which specific children were participating in the study and had no contact with the investigators. Thus, some potential for bias or influence was addressed but, importantly, Sam thought, not sufficiently focused on the play specialist's own potential for influence and interpretation. This section on reflexivity also requires consideration of how the researcher responded to events during the study and whether there were any changes in the research design. Other than extending the period of study (already discussed) the article made no reference to this aspect. Sam concluded that it is unlikely that any changes had been made, as it would surely have been mentioned. He did agree with Sue, however, that were he relying upon this evidence to change practice he would need to consult the primary data to be sure. Ethical issues are addressed in Question 7 and the extent to which these had been taken into consideration. Some detail was given of how the research was explained to the children and that they were under no pressure to participate. Issues of consent were also clearly addressed in the article but Sam could find no evidence to suggest that ethical permission had been sought from an appropriate NHS ethics committee. Sue and Sam had already discussed word constraints upon the authors but, notwithstanding this, decided this was an important omission on their part.

Data analysis

Data analysis was the next section and both Sue and Sam decided to tackle it together. Question 8 (with seven subsections) addressed this and asked whether the analysis was sufficiently rigorous. Subsections (a), (b) and (c) were straightforward to address: the article provided a reasonably in-depth description of the process of analysis, a thematic analysis *was* used and Riley's (1996) technique of coding data was used to delineate common themes. The researcher described how the data presented were selected from the original sample to demonstrate the analytical process. Subsection (d) asks whether there was sufficient data presented to support the findings. Despite the article being relatively short – just seven pages – Sue and Sam felt there was sufficient description to support the results. Two drawings by the same child were also reproduced in the article to illustrate their findings. Both Sam and Sue felt that here a picture painted a thousand words and that the reader could immediately follow the authors' claims. Neither Sue nor Sam, however, considered that the authors had completely satisfied the next two parts of the data analysis section. They both believed that there had been no discussion of contradictory data and no critical examination of bias or influence in the selection of data for presentation.

Research findings

Question 9 of the appraisal tool is concerned with the research findings and asks whether there was a clear statement of these. Sam had searched the article for a specific section headed 'findings' but it alluded him, although he deduced that this was contained in the discussion of results. On close reading he considered the findings were clear and explicit and supported by two tables. Some discussion of the credibility of the findings was included but there appeared to be no discussion of the evidence for and against the researchers' arguments, although the findings were contextualised with respect to the original research questions. The authors claimed that 'the results of this qualitative study of clown humour show that sick children believe that it is generally positive in ameliorating their fears and apprehensions about their hospital admission'. Sam thought this rather a bold statement given that only 20 children had been studied and thought that their claims should have been modified to reflect the localized nature of the study.

The value of the research

The final section (Question 10) asks how valuable the research is and whether the researcher discussed the contribution the study makes to existing knowledge or understanding. Sue was clear that the authors had claimed that the study added to the growing literature base for the efficacy of clown humour as experienced by children in hospital. She also reminded Sam that the limitations of the study were also identified and included that data were collected from children in only one hospital.

Reflection

When Sue and Sam reflected upon the process of critical appraisal they had undertaken they agreed that the research had some merits. They believed that the methodology was suitable for the nature of the enquiry and that the research had been conducted appropriately. The data collection was consistent with the methodological approach and addressed the research issue. They decided that the data analysis had also been conducted rigorously but that some important discussion points were missing from the article. One of the study's weakest areas appeared to Sue and Sam to be in the area of reflexivity. There seemed to have been little consideration of the relationship between researcher and participants and insufficient account made of the ethical considerations. On balance they concluded, as indeed the researchers had themselves, that further study was needed before any confidence could be given to the transferability of the findings or any change in practice made.

Having completed this exercise Sue and Sam discussed how they might write up the process and outcomes of their critical appraisal. They had been advised that where they had several articles using the same research methodology they should initially complete individual appraisals on each of the articles, but when they wrote them up they should compare each article section by section. So, for instance, if they had five articles using a qualitative methodology, they should discuss all of them with respect to their satisfying the screening questions, and then the research design for each of them, and so on. They both felt more able to approach the task now and decided to make a start on appraising the qualitative articles they had found from their literature search and to structure their summaries according to the sections of the appraisal tool. They could see that this process would give them plenty of material for the 'discussion' section of their dissertations as they would be able to comment upon the relative strengths and weaknesses of each of the articles. This process would enable them to decide on balance whether there was enough 'good research' to support a change in practice.

References

Greenhalgh, T. (2010) *How to Read a Paper* (4th edn). Blackwell Publishing, London.

NHS (2012) Critical Appraisal Skills Programme. http://www.sph.nhs.uk/what-we-do/public-health-workforce/resources/critical-appraisals-skills-programme (accessed 24 May 2012).

Public Health Resource Unit (2006) Critical Appraisal Skills Programme: 10 Questions to help you make sense of Qualitative Research. Public Health Resource Unit, England. http://www.sph.nhs.uk/sph-files/Qualitative%20Appraisal%20Tool.pdf (accessed 11 February 2011).

Riley, J. (1996) *Getting the most form your data. A handbook of practical ideas on how to analyse qualitative data.* Technical and Educational Services Ltd.

Weaver, K., Prudhoe, G., Battrick, C. And Glasper, E.A. (2007) Sick children's perceptions of clown doctor humour. *British Journal of Nursing*, **1** (8), 359–365.

For further resources for this chapter visit the companion website at

🖳 **www.wiley.com/go/glasper/nursingdissertation**

Chapter 17   Critically reviewing quantitative papers using a CASP critiquing tool

Steve George
University of Southampton, UK

Activity

From your university online library provision source and print the journal paper: Lattimer, V., George, S., Thompson, F. *et al.* (1998) General Practice. Safety and effectiveness of nurse telephone consultation in out of hour's primary care: randomised controlled trial. *British Medical Journal*, **317**, 1054–1059.

(Chapters 16 and 17 gives more information on CASP.)

Download from the CASP website a copy of the randomised controlled trial appraisal tool (http://www.casp-uk.net/).

Use your highlighter pens to follow the narrative in this chapter.

Scenario

Sam and Sue have been asked by their supervisors to critique an empirical paper by using one of the CASP critiquing tools. The paper is based on a Randomised Controlled Trial and Sue is worried about the amount of data within the paper. She is overawed by the questions posed within the critiquing tool and over coffee she and Sam confer. Sam has come across a *British Medical Journal* paper by Lattimer *et al.* (1998) and he uses this to help explain how to use the CASP critiquing tool.

SUE: 'Sam, this is really difficult. I don't even know what some of the questions mean, let alone the answers to them. Why does it have to be so complicated?'

How to Write Your Nursing Dissertation, First Edition. Alan Glasper and Colin Rees.
© 2013 John Wiley & Sons, Ltd. Published 2013 by John Wiley & Sons, Ltd.

166

SAM: 'It isn't complicated really Sue. What the CASP scheme does is to break down what is potentially a complex question into easily answerable bits. Come on, let's have a go'

Question 1 'Did the study ask a clearly-focused question?'

SUE: 'Why is that important to ask as the first question? Aren't there more important things?'

SAM: 'No, the reason is that if the answer's 'No' you can stop reading at that point! If they haven't asked a clearly focused question they're not going to get an answer which means anything. So let's look at the question they've asked in this paper. Actually, they've phrased it as an objective. Their objective was:

To determine the safety and effectiveness of nurse telephone consultation in out of hours primary care by investigating adverse events and the management of calls.'

SUE: 'Is that clearly focused enough?'

SAM: 'Well, what do you think?'

SUE: 'It sounds OK to me, but what do I know about it?'

SAM: 'It sounds OK to me too. If you look at what they've published previously they undertook a survey of General Practitioner opinion a couple of years earlier, in which it became clear that the 'safety' of putting nurses on the telephone to answer patients' calls was a concern amongst GPs at that time. It follows that a sensible aim of a large scale study looking at nurse telephone consultation would be to establish its safety, and if they're going to do that it makes sense to do a study of effectiveness at the same time.'

SUE: 'I saw that they'd done the GP survey but then I noticed that they'd also done a pilot study previously. Why didn't they do the safety study at that stage?'

SAM: 'People often ask that. Generally speaking, when you're looking at the outcome of trials, the 'effectiveness' outcomes are far more common than the 'adverse event' outcomes by which we measure safety. In order to get to the adverse events we have to collect data on a large number of people – many more than would be included in a pilot study. Pilot studies are fine for establishing that the intervention will actually work (meaning that you can run it, not that it will be effective) and that the intervention will be acceptable, but not for establishing safety. In fact, many randomised controlled trials, even drug trials, don't look at safety – that's established much later by post-marketing surveillance studies. OK, you can rule out obvious toxicity early on in phase 1 and phase 2 trials, but not some of the rare side effects. You can look at effectiveness within a trial designed to measure safety, but not necessarily the other way around, because the numbers might not be enough.'

SUE: 'Hang on, hang on! Phase what?'

SAM: 'Sorry, getting a bit technical, but this is important stuff. Drug trials are classified into four types, generally speaking. Phase 1 trials are studies of small doses of new compounds in healthy volunteers and phase 2 trials are initial clinical studies in disease sufferers with the aim of establishing whether it's worth proceeding to a full scale trial. Phase 3 trials, often incorporating analysis of things like cost effectiveness of a new intervention, are the ones we generally think about as randomised controlled trials, and phase 4 trials aren't really trials at all: they're post-marketing surveillance studies designed to look at safety, usually of drugs, and including thousands of people.'

SUE: 'OK, so this is a phase 3 trial then?'

SAM: 'Yes, although safety was its primary outcome. The pharmaceutical terminology isn't used so often in non-drug intervention studies like this, and most non-drug trials are phase 3, although there's quite a case to be made for more early-phase studies of non-drug interventions. You might want to look at the Medical Research Council's guidance on developing and evaluating complex interventions, the last version of which came out in 2008. It's on their website.'

SUE: 'Right, I'll do that. What about the next question?'

Question 2   'Was this a randomised controlled trial (RCT) and was it appropriately so?'

SUE: 'I get mixed up over this. You see, all of these people telephoned in, didn't they? They're not a random sample of the population at all.'

SAM: 'This is another one people often get wrong. Subjects in a randomised controlled trial *aren't* randomly selected from the population. There wouldn't be any point in doing that. If you were going to test a new antihypertensive drug you'd want all the subjects in your trial to have high blood pressure, and if you randomly selected them from the population they wouldn't. No, subjects in a randomised controlled trial are often highly selected, and "random", in this case, refers to the method by which you allocate them to treatment within the trial, not the means by which you select them from the population.'

SUE: 'Oh, I see. So "random" isn't about selection? That actually makes more sense. I'm looking at how they did the randomisation though, and it doesn't look like what I've seen before. Whenever I've looked at trials it seemed to be that patients were admitted to the trial, had their details taken, signed a consent form and were then given either one treatment or the other. But that's not what happened here is it?'

SAM: 'No, it isn't, but you've got to look at the way in which the intervention was set up and consider the alternatives. In order to do what you've just described the investigators would have had to have set up two services, one using nurses on the telephone, one not, working in parallel, at the same time, and sent each patient to one of them or the other. That would have been very costly to do, if not logistically impossible. So they did what was possible and split the year up into periods when the nurse service ran and periods when it didn't.'

SUE: 'But is that random? How did they randomise?'

SAM: 'They used a method called "block randomisation". This is often done in drug trials in order to iron out differences in numbers of subjects in each arm of a trial. Rather than using a completely random sequence of numbers the trial is divided into blocks of four or six subjects, commonly, and within each block two (of four) or three (of six) subjects are allocated to each intervention. Allocation within each block is random, so the whole sequence of all the blocks placed one after another becomes random.'

SUE: 'But why not just use a random sequence of numbers?'

SAM: 'Because it can result in quite considerable differences of numbers in different arms of trials, particularly if a trial is small. I remember well a student pilot trial in which they only intended to recruit 20 patients. The trouble is, they used a simple random sequence and ended up with 19 people in one arm and only one in the other. Essentially it meant that the study was useless! That can't happen with blocked randomisation'

SUE: 'That sounds like a good idea then. But does blocked randomisation ever lead to problems?'

SAM: 'It can do, in that if it is known that a trial is block randomised in, say, blocks of four, it becomes possible to predict to which group the last case in a block is allocated. A clinician wishing to push a patient into one treatment group or another might, therefore, be able to move patients around to get their chosen patient into their preferred group. You get around that by using a mixture of blocks of different sizes, say four and six, so it becomes impossible to predict.'

SUE: 'And how did they do it in this study?'

SAM: 'They used a method I'd not seen before – in fact, it might have been the first time it had been used. They divided the year over which they were going to run the trial into a series of twenty six blocks of two weeks. Within each block they therefore had two Monday evenings, two Tuesday evenings, two weekends and so on. They then randomised so that one or other of the two became a period during which the service ran. Each one of those evenings or weekends became an allocation unit within the trial, with the patients ringing in during that block allocated to one service or the other. They obtained consent on behalf of the patients from the participating general practitioners.'

SUE: 'So this is a phase 3 block randomised controlled trial? How do I tell whether or not the randomisation was appropriate?'

SAM: 'There are two questions here – firstly, was a randomised trial the appropriate way of answering this question and, secondly, whether the way in which it was done was appropriate. You'll have seen the Cochrane Hierarchy of Evidence?'

SUE: 'Yes, and it puts the randomised controlled trial nearly at the top of the evidence tree. They call it "the gold standard" for research.'

SAM: 'Yes, that's right, but it's the gold standard only for the question *"How effective (or safe) is a new treatment in the management of a specified ailment compared to a placebo or to the best existing treatment?"* For other questions other research designs are better. A randomised controlled trial won't answer the question "What is the cause of this rare disease?", and it won't tell you why patients don't like, say, turning up to antenatal clinics. The first of those questions is best addressed by a case-control study and the second by, most likely, a qualitative study in the first instance, possibly followed up by a survey designed using data from the qualitative study. Even in the case of effectiveness of an intervention a single randomised controlled trial is bettered by a systematic review of several well designed randomised controlled trials. However, in this case, a randomised controlled trial was the best way to answer the question set, and there hadn't been a previous trial on this subject with which it could be included in a systematic review.'

SUE: 'Fine, I understand that now. And did they do it appropriately?'

Question 3 'Were participants appropriately allocated to intervention and control groups?'

SAM: 'Well, you can look at what they did, but the best way to tell if randomisation has been effective is to look at the tables of baseline data for a trial – often Table 1, but in this paper split between Tables 2 and 3. As a broad rule, if the two groups randomised are broadly similar randomisation has worked, and if they're not, it hasn't.'

SUE: 'It looks as if it worked in this case then.'

SAM: 'I would say so. The numbers in each group overall are similar and there are only a few minor differences between numbers in different age groups, which I doubt influenced results in any important fashion. If there *had* been differences it would have been important to look at how participants were allocated to the intervention and control groups, whether the process was truly random, whether the method of allocation was described, whether any method was used to balance the randomization, like stratification, how the randomization schedule was generated and how a participant was allocated to a study group. Now, what about blinding?'

Question 4 'Were participants, staff and study personnel 'blind' to participants study group?'

SUE: 'I find blinding a difficult subject. Perhaps I'm just stupid.'

SAM: 'Nonsense – the reason you find it difficult is that it *is* difficult, more so than some people realise. When you're assessing blinding you not only have to think about whether blinding was absent or present but also who was blinded and who wasn't, and what the potential effect of non-blinding would be in each case. And people also fail to separate "blinding" from "allocation concealment", which can have different effects on a trial. You also have to consider, if you're ever going to conduct a trial, what you can do to minimise the effects of non-blinding.'

SUE: 'Go on, remind me about blinding …'

SAM: 'Tutorial coming up! A blinded trial is one in which the design prevents participants, carers or those assessing outcome from knowing which intervention group a participant was in. Blinding is sometimes impossible, for instance in trials of surgical operations – ethically "sham procedures", in which a patient ends up with the external signs of having had an operation in the form of a scar but where no procedure was performed, are frowned upon. Also, trials of therapies involving active patient participation – like "talking therapies" or physiotherapy, can't be blinded easily.'

SUE: 'And what about "single blind" and "double blind" trials?'

SAM: 'I'm glad you asked that, but it's really historical now. Various studies reported that different authors used those terms – and also used "triple blind" – but meant different things by the terms. For instance, some authors used "single blind" to mean that subjects in the trial were blinded to what they were getting but those running the trial or assessing the outcome weren't, but others used it to mean exactly the opposite. The 2010 CONSORT Statement recommended that the use of these terms was terminated and that reports of trials which were meant to be blinded should discuss, instead "If done, who was blinded after assignment to interventions (for example, participants, care providers, those assessing outcomes) and how?"'

SUE: 'And what about the effects of non-blinding?'

SAM: 'Well the main effect of non-blinding is primarily on assessment of outcomes, and so the magnitude of the effect depends on how subjective, or not, an outcome is. A patient in a trial of an agent designed to help them stop smoking might be more inclined to report that they've stopped if they know they've had the active intervention. Likewise, a researcher assessing a patient and who knew they'd been on the active intervention might be more inclined to report a favourable outcome because they have a vested interest in finding one. However, if you have a blood test to tell you whether or not they've been smoking that is much less subjective and so non-blinding doesn't matter so much.'

SUE: 'I can't see how they might have blinded this trial.'

SAM: 'No, and they don't claim to have blinded it. It's pretty obvious whether or not you spoke straightaway to a doctor or whether or not you spoke to a nurse first, or only to a nurse. But the outcomes were all pretty objective, total deaths, got from death certificates, and numbers of A&E attendances and hospital admissions, so it's unlikely to matter that it wasn't blinded. But while we're on the subject let's talk about "allocation concealment", which is the procedure for protecting the randomisation process so that the treatment to be allocated is not known before a patient is entered into the study. In this case the pattern of intervention was known only to the lead investigators throughout the study. Nurses and doctors working on the ground were blind to the intervention until a point when they would be unable to choose or swap duty periods, so, for instance, a doctor couldn't decide that they weren't going to work on a night when the nurse service was working, or not. The doctor or nurse pattern was not publicised anywhere and only became apparent to members of the public on the day of calling.'

SUE: 'So is that enough?'

SAM: 'In the context of this trial I think it's the best that could be done. Right, onwards and upwards! Next question.'

Question 5   'Were all of the participants who entered the trial accounted for at its conclusion?'

SUE: 'Doesn't that always happen?'

SAM: 'No, it doesn't, unfortunately. It's always worth checking. Have you heard of "Intention to Treat Analysis (ITT)"?'

SUE: 'Vaguely...'

SAM: 'Mmm. Well, people vary in the way in which they interpret the term. In order to do ITT analysis properly you need to account for *every* person who was recruited to the trial and make sure they were analysed in the group to which they were first assigned, not the one in which they ended up – which in drug trials can be different for various reasons – and that they're not left out because, for instance, they didn't complete the course of treatment. In this trial people were entered according to the system in operation at the time they called, so swapping groups isn't really an option, and all the tables add up, so nobody's been left out of the analysis. Next question...'

Question 6   'Were the participants in all groups followed up and data collected in the same way?'

SUE: 'I've looked at this and I can't see that they were treated differently in any way.'

SAM: 'I would say that they were treated the same way. The investigators seem to have collected data on workload from the database of calls, data on mortality from the Office For National Statistics, data on admissions from local hospitals and then data on attendance at A&E from GP cooperative records, all using the total list of names and addresses of people that called, and they then matched the data gathered to the period in which they called, so it would have been difficult to treat them differently.'

SUE: 'And how about Question 7?'

Question 7   **Did the study have enough participants to minimise the play of chance?'**

SAM: 'Well from your point of view the first thing to look out for is that they've done a sample size calculation before starting the trial. Then, look to see if they actually achieved that sample size during recruitment. In this trial they did both, so I'd give that box a tick. Statisticians use specialist software to calculate sample sizes and unless it's something quite simple you're unlikely to be able to replicate the calculation by yourself. So, unless you're planning on becoming a statistician and spending quite a lot of money on software, I'd leave it at that! Question 8 then…'

Question 8   **'How are the results presented and what is the main result?'**

SAM: 'OK. What did they find?'

SUE: 'I found this difficult as well, because they say this is an equivalence trial, and I'd never heard of one of those'.

SAM: 'Yes, equivalence trials are a subject area all to themselves. But they're not that hard once you know the basics. The first part to get around is that you can't prove that two treatments have exactly the same effect.'

SUE: 'Why not?'

SAM: 'Because in order to do that you'd need an infinite number of people in each arm of the trial. And that's not just one infinite number of people, that's two infinite numbers of people!'

SUE: 'Oh, so what do you do then?'

SAM: 'You have to specify a range within which you believe that a difference in clinical effect is of no importance. There are various ways of doing that, which seem to range from just pulling a number out of a hat to looking at looking at patient estimates of whether an effect is important. That's particularly useful when you're looking at patient reported outcomes. A lot depends on being able to specify the "minimal important clinical difference". This can be done using information gathered from previous papers, or from pilot studies.'

SUE: 'And what about this paper?'

SAM: 'They looked at the existing death rate for England and calculated an expected number of deaths based on the size of the population covered by the GP cooperative used for the trial – that in itself is quite a small number of deaths. They then set limits around it from 80 to 125% of that number, which is a range used in bioequivalence studies.'

SUE: 'So to show equivalence they just had to show a number of deaths between those limits?'

SAM: 'Not quite – they had to show a number of deaths *plus the confidence intervals around it* between the equivalence limits. And those confidence intervals are the key to understanding equivalence trials, and why they tend to be much bigger than trials designed to show a difference.'

SUE: 'Go on...'

SAM: 'You see, everybody wants to specify the narrowest pair of equivalence limits they can, but in order to do that you need to get a very narrow confidence interval around whatever you're measuring as the outcome of the trial, and trying to achieve a narrower confidence always means getting more people into the study.'

SUE: 'I see. And they did show equivalence I see. What would have happened if they hadn't? Would they have been able to say that the two interventions were different?'

SAM: 'Not necessarily. They might have, but only if the area covered by the confidence intervals lay completely outside the area defined by the equivalence limits. If the confidence intervals crossed either equivalence limit they'd have had to have said that they were uncertain whether there was equivalence or not.'

SUE: 'And that would mean that there was no statistically significant difference?'

SAM: 'Again, not necessarily. They could have a statistically significant difference, because the confidence intervals did not include the line of no difference. But if it crossed one of the equivalence limits, the difference, although significant, might not be important. And statistical significance and clinical importance aren't the same thing.'

SUE: 'But when you see difference trials reported they usually just tell you about the significant result they've got.'

SAM: 'Quite true. In that way equivalence trials are more honest than difference trials, because you have to state at the outset when you're planning your trial and what you consider to be important differences, whereas, as you say, difference trials often don't tell you at all whether they think the difference they've found is important.'

SUE: 'And is that what they did for all the outcomes?'

SAM: 'Yes, they did, with equivalence limits and confidence intervals, and confidence intervals bring us onto the next question.'

Question 9   'How precise are these results?'

SUE: 'Haven't we just done that?'

SAM: 'We have, but in a difference trial we might by now have looked at the magnitude of the result but not at the confidence intervals around it.'

SUE: 'And can we make a decision using the results we've seen?'

SAM: 'Well I think we ought to move onto the final question before answering that…'

Question 10   'Were all important outcomes considered so the results can be applied?'

SUE: 'I think that they did consider all the important outcomes. Let's see, they looked at deaths within seven days of a contact with the out of hours service, emergency hospital admissions within 24 hours and within three days of contact, attendance at accident and emergency within three days of a contact and how all the calls were managed and by whom. Isn't that enough?'

SAM: 'Yes, I think it is. But what you've got to ask is "What decision am I being asked to make?" This trial was the first one to look at the safety of nurse telephone consultation services and as far as I'm aware the only one to date. But the results have to be looked at in light of the service being tested. In this trial the nurses worked within the context of a primary care cooperative, and they haven't existed since the change in the GP contract a few years ago removed GPs' responsibility for out of hours care. So, the result showing that calls needing to be handled by doctors were reduced by 50% can't now be interpreted, unless a similar system comes into operation again. One of the major problems with randomised controlled trials is that their results are too often applied to people who weren't represented in the trial population, or in circumstances which are different from those pertaining in the trial.'

SUE: 'Oh. So is there nothing we can learn from this trial any more?'

SAM: 'I'm not saying that. The major concern prior to the trial was about the safety of nurses undertaking telephone consultation and that result still stands. But the results of this trial were used by the government to inform the setting up of NHS Direct, which wasn't linked to primary care and, consequently, never showed the reduction in workload for out of hours medical care.'

SUE: 'OK. That's an important lesson. Thanks Sam.'

For further resources for this chapter visit the companion website at
   www.wiley.com/go/glasper/nursingdissertation

Chapter 18 Critically reviewing a journal paper using the Parahoo model

Kader Parahoo[1] and Irene Heuter[2]
[1]*University of Ulster, UK*
[2]*Columbia University, New York, USA*

Scenario

Sue and Sam are investigating which critiquing tool to use for the analysis of their selected scholarly papers. Sam has read some of the work of Professor Kader Parahoo, who is Professor of Nursing research at the University of Ulster. They are interested in using his model of critiquing, which is discussed in more detail in this chapter.

Introduction

Evidence-based practice depends, amongst other things, on researchers providing robust evidence from their studies. To decide whether a study has been rigorously carried out and whether its findings are relevant for your practice, you need to develop critical appraisal skills. The terms 'appraisal' or 'evaluation' of a published research paper are often used interchangeably to refer to the process of judging the quality of a study and its relevance for one's practice.

Activity

Use your university online learning environment to access this paper. You should be able to download a fully copy free of charge: Rice, M., Glasper, A., Keeton, D. and Spargo, P. (2008) The effect of a preoperative education programme on perioperative anxiety in children: an observational study. *Pediatric Anesthesia*, **18**, 426–430.
   Use your highlighter pens to help you in the process of critiquing this paper.

How to Write Your Nursing Dissertation, First Edition. Alan Glasper and Colin Rees.
© 2013 John Wiley & Sons, Ltd. Published 2013 by John Wiley & Sons, Ltd.

Framework for appraisal

There are many tools for appraising or evaluating research studies (e.g. SIGN, 2009; ScHARR, 2009). In this chapter, the framework provided by Parahoo (2006:Chapter 17, Evaluating Research Studies) will be used to appraise the Rice *et al.* (2008) paper. The framework consists of the following headings, which are based on the structure that is most often used to report quantitative studies in research journals. The headings are:

- Title of study
- Abstract
- Literature review/Background
- Methodology or Design
- Results
- Discussion and interpretation (including limitations)
- Recommendations

Title of study

Does the title convey the study clearly and accurately?

> The title of this paper reflects a study that tests the effects of a preoperative education programme (independent variable) on preoperative anxiety (dependent variable) in children (the population). Therefore, the title contains all the key components in this study (the variables, the type of relationship between them, i.e. 'effect', and the population). The title also identifies the design of the study (observational).

From the title can I decide whether this paper is relevant to my practice?

> If I work in paediatric care where induction of anaesthesia is carried out, then this study is highly relevant to me.

Abstract

Does the abstract give a short and concise summary of the following aspects of the study?

- *Background*
  The study is put in context by pointing out the distress and potential harm to children who have to receive anaesthesia. Some of the strategies used to minimise anxiety in children are mentioned and the authors briefly state that a Saturday Morning Club (SMC) has been in existence at their own hospital to address this issue.

- *Aim*
  The aim was 'to assess the influence of attendance at a Saturday Morning Club (the preoperative education programme) on anxiety in patients of age between 2 and 16 years'.

- *Designs*
  An observational study design was used in this study. Patient anxiety was measured by the modified Preoperative Anxiety Scale; parental anxiety was self-reported and assessed by means of a visual analogue scale. The assessment time points were on the day ward, in the preoperative waiting room and at induction of anaesthesia.

  The sample comprised 94 children aged between 2 and 16 years old. Twenty-one attended the SMC and 73 did not. We are told that observers were unaware (blinded) of who had attended or not. There is also mention of the statistical test: the Mann-Whitney U-test.

- *Results*
  The results are briefly and clearly presented. Attendance was reported as having had a 'favourable effect' on patient anxiety, but that this was only statistically significant in the waiting room. However, the results for parental anxiety were not given in the abstract.

- *Conclusions*
  Further studies are recommended to provide evidence to support the use of a preoperative education programme. However, the authors do not comment on the evidence produced by this study.

  Overall the abstract is well written and presented. It is a very good example of how an abstract can be short and yet provide readers with relevant information for them to decide whether the study has some merit and is worth reading.

Literature review/Background

- *Is the importance of study justified?*
  The authors justify the importance of this study by identifying (in the first four sentences of the introduction) the main stress-related problems associated with the induction of anaesthesia in children. Relevant studies are appropriately referenced. Some of the problems listed are: physiological, physical and psychological. The authors mention nightmares, eating disorders, enuresis and behavioural problems. The link between parental anxiety and children's distress is also briefly mentioned.

- *What is the context of this study?*
  This study was carried out to investigate the effect of an existing preoperative educational programme (in the form of a Saturday Morning Club) on children about to undergo day case surgery. The programme is itself briefly described. The information given is adequate for readers to understand what the programme entails.

- *Does the literature review show the gap(s) in knowledge which this study seeks to fill?*

With reference to the literature, the authors list the main strategies used to reduce anxiety. These include premedication, parental presence at induction, psychological preparation and preoperative education (leaflets, books or play therapy). There is no indication of whether all or any of these have an effect on children's anxiety. However, in the discussion section, we are informed that 'several studies have demonstrated the efficacy of premedication' (p. 428). The authors state in the discussion that 'preoperative education programmes are costly' and that 'evidence of their benefit is variable' (p. 428). It would have been helpful if this information was provided in the introduction.

Presumably the 'Saturday Morning Club' is the first of its kind (but we are not told this in the introduction).

Aims/objectives/research questions/hypotheses

- *Are the aims of the study clear?*
  The main aim of the study is clear (see the last sentence under Introduction). The study investigated the effect of the education programme on anxiety in children undergoing day care surgery. There is, however, no mention of the other aim, which is to measure parental anxiety as well. At this stage it is not clear if the authors intend to assess the relationship between children's distress and parental anxiety.

Design of study

- *What is the design of the study? Is it the most appropriate for the aims of the study?*
  A prospective observational study design was selected. The NIH (2009) defines observational study as one

'in which the investigators do not manipulate the use of, or deliver, an intervention (e.g. do not assign patients to treatment and control groups), but only observe patients who are (and sometimes patients who are not as a basis of comparison) exposed to the intervention, and interpret the outcomes'.

This type of design is appropriate for evaluating the effects of an intervention or practice which was already in place. Under 'limitations of study', the authors explain that it was thought 'to be unethical to conduct an RCT' as the SMC was 'an established facility' in the hospital.

This study is prospective because the participants were 'followed' from the time they attended the SMC (two weeks before surgery) to the time they came for elective surgery.

The strength of an observational study is that researchers do not seek to manipulate the situation (i.e. change normal practice to carry out the experiment). Instead, in observational studies, researchers study real-life situations.

In an observational study, researchers do not have control over the selection and allocation of participants to groups. For example, in this case an SMC was already offered to parents and children who decided to attend or not. Observational studies are, therefore, prone to selection bias. For this reason the evidence from observational studies is not considered to be as strong as that from good randomised controlled trials (RCTs).

Observational studies can, however, 'indicate' whether an intervention works and this can be further tested by RCTs (as recommended by the authors of this study).

- *Are the main concepts (to be measured) defined?*

The main concept measured is the 'distress' (DAI) of children. No operational definition of 'distress' is given but an Anxiety Scale is used to measure distress. One could ask if 'distress' and 'anxiety' can be used interchangeably.

- *What are the methods of data collection? Are they constructed for the purpose of the current study or do the researchers use existing ones?*

The main instrument used in this study is the 'modified Yale Preoperative Anxiety Scale' (mYPAS) to measure anxiety in children preoperatively and at induction of anaesthesia. Parental anxiety was self-reported using a 100 mm visual analogue scale (VAS).

The use of the Yale Preoperative Anxiety Scale (YPAS) was justified because 'it is sensitive to changes in anxiety over time' and it has 'good inter-observer reliability and high construct concurrent validity' (p. 427). What is not clear, however, is who modified the YPAS. Was it the researchers in this study? Or was there a modified version? If the latter, there is no reference for it. If the former, why was it modified and how does this affect the internal consistency of the original YPAS?

The justification for the use of the VAS for measuring parental anxiety was because it 'is widely used and has good validity when compared with other assessment methods' (p. 429).

- *Who collected data? Can this introduce bias in the study?*

To avoid observation bias, two observers who were blinded to the study were used (i.e. they did not know who participated in the SMC or not).

To minimise observation errors and achieve a degree of consistency between the two observers, a pilot study was performed to assess inter-observer reliability. The Kappa test 'showed excellent agreement between the two observers' scores' (p. 427).

- *In studies where there is more than one group, is there a description of what intervention/treatment each group receives?*

In this study both groups (SMC attenders and non-attenders) received the same care and treatment, although the anaesthetist and anaesthetic management were not standardised. In a study of real-life situations (as in this case) it is neither practical nor ethical to interfere with the care and treatment which the health service provides for patients.

The data collected for the two groups (demographic details, use of sedatives etc.) were well described.

• *Is the setting(s) where the study is carried out adequately described?*
The setting, procedures and policies were all adequately described. This information helps the reader to understand the context of the study and to compare with their own settings (in case they want to introduce the SMC at their own hospital).

• *Who was selected? From what population were they selected? What was the precise method of selection and allocation? Was there a sample size calculation?*
As explained earlier, in observational studies researchers have little control over the selection and allocation of participants to groups. In this study participants were recruited on the day of surgery. Every child who came for treatment was observed (whether they participated previously in the SMC or not. Only those 'who did not speak English as a first language and those who had severe developmental delay' (p. 427) were excluded.
There is no information about the target population. For example, while we are told that only 25% of families chose to attend the SMC, there is no indication of how many families attended the SMC monthly or annually.

Their rationale for the sample size (n = 94) is not given, although (in the limitations) the author expressed the view that it was 'not possible to state with any degree of certainty what reduction in the mYPAS scores would be clinically significant' and that was the reason why 'a power analysis was not undertaken' (p. 429). It also was not noted which mYPAS score range is considered to represent 'moderate' or 'severe' anxiety. Such a classification could have been employed in a sample size estimation.

• *Was ethical approval obtained? Are there any other ethical implications?*
Ethical approval was obtained from the institutional ethics committee. Informed consent was obtained from parents and children. As there is no mention of refusal from any parent or child, we can only assume that they all agreed to participate.

Those whose first language was not English and those with 'severe developmental delay' were excluded. It is possible that these two groups may have greater anxiety because of communication problems. Their needs should also be taken into account through research.

Data analysis

Was there a separate section in the paper that explained the planned analyses prior to the presentation of the results?

We are only told in the results section which statistical methods were used and how they were applied to the data. Most of this information can be gathered in the four separate tables that summarise (i) patient demographic data, (ii) patient baseline characteristics, (iii) patients anxiety scores by attenders/non-attenders and (iv) parental anxiety visual analogue scores by attenders/non-attenders.

- *Which statistical methods were relied on?*
  Generally, continuous variables, such as age, patient anxiety scores and parental anxiety visual analogue scores, were summarised by the median and interquartile range. The Mann-Whitney U-test was used to compare these variables between the two groups of SMC attenders and non-attenders. Categorical variables, such as number of male patients and number of patients who previously had general anaesthesia, were summarised by frequency counts and percentages. The Fisher exact test was used to compare categorical variables between the two groups of SMC attenders and non-attenders. P-values are determined to be statistically significant if they do not exceed 0.05.

  It is suitable to list the median and interquartile range as summary statistics for the variables that are analysed via the Mann-Whitney U-test, because this is a non-parametric test and compares the difference in the medians of the two groups. The column header of Table 1 that says 'Kruskal Wallis test' is a bit confusing. Firstly, since there are two groups, the header should have stated 'Mann-Whitney U-test'. Secondly, it is not clear how the 'Kruskal Wallis test' could have been applied to the categorical variables 'Total number of SMC attenders' and 'Number of male patients'.

- *Is it clear how the statistical tests were applied to the data and groups?*
  The table presentation clearly identifies the variables, groups, statistical tests performed and the resulting test results (here, p-values). It is easy for the reader to follow.

Results

- *Are the results clearly presented?*
  The results in the text and in the tables are clearly presented.

  As usual for this type of study, the demographic details and other parameters, such as previous history of general anaesthesia, method of anaesthesia, parental presence at induction, use of premedication and so on, are provided. This allows readers to assess whether the two groups were similar in these respects.

- *Are the results for all the aims presented?*
  The aims were to measure patient and parent anxiety. The results of both these aims are provided.

- *Are the results fully presented?*
  In addition to the results stated about the statistical significance of the group comparisons at each time point, one could have mentioned a noticeable increasing trend in the anxiety levels in the SMC non-attenders group for both patients and parents, which is much less emphasised in the SMC attenders group. For example, the medians stay or nearly stay the same in the waiting area as in the day ward for the SMC attenders, while the same medians markedly increase for the SMC non-attenders.

Discussion

Most of the statements under the 'Discussion' section are about the variety of methods to address anxiety associated with anaesthesia and their effectiveness. Most of this should have been in the introduction/background. The 'real' discussion, in this study is under the heading 'Limitations'.

- *Is it a balanced discussion? Have all possible explanations for the results been given?*
  Overall, it is a well-balanced discussion. The authors offer a number of ways to interpret the results. However, they did not elaborate as to why they think a type II error could account for the failure to detect a statistically significant difference between the score of the two groups on the day ward and in the anaesthetic room.
- *Are the results discussed in the context of previous studies?*
  The design and findings of a number of relevant studies were discussed in an attempt to put the findings of this study in the context of what is already known on this topic. Readers are therefore provided with information on other similar studies to follow up, if they wish.
- *Are the results fully discussed?*
  While the authors mention that the 'present study has shown that children who have attended our preadmission education programme (the SMC) have statistically significant lower anxiety levels in the waiting area than those who have not attended the SMC', this finding has not been leveraged against the findings that SMC non-attenders generally were older and had previously had anaesthesia. This could have impacted the results based on statistical inference in either way if these factors were incorporated in the analysis. We do not know.

  It is mentioned in the 'Limitations' later on that possibly the older children in this study, who are also more likely to have received a previous general anaesthetic, have already attended the SMC. This remains speculation, since unfortunately the number of patients who previously attended SMC and the number of patients who previously had general anaesthetic were not recorded in this study. This is somewhat of a shortcoming of this study and should be built in in any future (randomised) trial.

- *Are the limitations of the study discussed?*
  The authors pointed out that it was not possible to conduct an RCT and gave reasons for this. They also admitted that no data were recorded on whether some of the older children had received a previous general anaesthetic or may have attended the SMC on an earlier occasion.

  Another limitation which the authors identified is that they did not take into account that the relationship between the timing of the programme (SMC) and the age of children, as younger children may have shorter recall times.

Conclusions/Recommendations

- *Are the conclusions justified?*
  The authors are justified in claiming that the results show their programme (attendance at the SMC) reduced patient anxiety in the waiting area. The design of the study is robust enough for readers to reach this conclusion.
- *Are there recommendations for policy, practice or further research?*
  The authors recommended a larger RCT to examine the cost-effectiveness of this programme in the United Kingdom setting.
  They could also have recommended that future studies include those whose primary language is not English and also other vulnerable groups, such as children with physical and/or mental disability, where possible.
- *Are the results/conclusions helpful for my practice?*
  In the absence of more robust evidence, I would use the findings of this study (less anxiety among those who attended the SMC, especially in the waiting area) to inform my practice. Evidence-based practice takes into account the following:
  - Evidence from research
  - Clinical expertise
  - Patients' preferences and wishes
  (Sackett et al., 1996)

  My decision will also take into account the cost of the SMC. Although all these factors are important, the findings of this study will increase my confidence if I am contemplating the possibility of implementing such a programme.
- *Are the results generalisable?*
  The results are not generalisable to all children, since those who attended the SMC were self-selective. Only 25% of those offered the SMC attended. Among these, it is not clear which age group benefitted the most. In this study the ages of children ranged from 2 to 16. Being at different developmental stages, it is unlikely that such programmes may affect these children in the same way. Further analysis of the data and future research could shed more light on the effects of such programmes on younger and older children.

Funding

- *Is there potential conflict of interest (if information on funding is provided)?*
No information on who funded this study is provided.

Conclusion

This study seemed to have served its purpose by providing information on whether anxiety at induction was influenced by attendance at a SMC two weeks previously. In some ways one could describe it as a pilot study (e.g. the sample was quite small) which raised a number of questions that could be more rigorously investigated by a large randomised controlled trial. Nonetheless, the quality of this study itself is good enough for the findings to be taken seriously.

References

NIH (National Institute of Health) (2009) http//www.nlm.nih.gov/nichsr/hta101/ta101014.html (accessed 15 September 2009).

Parahoo, K. (2006) *Nursing Research: Principles, Process and Issues* (2nd edn). Palgrave, Basingstoke.

Rice, M., Glasper, A., Keeton, D. and Spargo, P. (2008) The effect of a preoperative education programme on perioperative anxiety in children: an observational study. *Pediatric Anesthesia*, **18**, 426–430.

Sackett, D.L., Rosenberg, W.M.C., Muir Gray, J.A., Haynes, R.B. and Richardson, W.S. (1996) Evidence based medicine: What it is and what it isn't. *British Medical Journal*, **312**, 71–72.

ScHARR (School of Health and Related Research) (2009) http://www.shef.ac.uk/scharr/ (accessed on 5 October 2009).

SIGN (Scottish Intercollegiate Guidelines Network) (2009) http://www.sign.ac.uk/methodology/checklists.html (accessed on 5 October 2009).

For further resources for this chapter visit the companion website at
www.wiley.com/go/glasper/nursingdissertation

Chapter 19 Critically reviewing a journal paper using the Rees model

Alan Glasper[1] and Colin Rees[2]
[1]*University of Southampton, UK*
[2]*University of Cardiff, UK*

Scenario

Sam wants to practice using the critiquing framework by Rees (2011). He has an article by Ellis and Glasper (2007) and wants to use this as a way of helping him prepare for critically evaluating research papers. He plans to share this with his supervisor to ensure that he has understood and can explain the different elements in a study. In particular, he wants to ensure he can differentiate between a quantitative and qualitative study from the way it is presented, especially where it is not straightforward, as in this study, where the technique of data collection is unfamiliar.

Activity

Use your university online learning environment to access the paper: Ellis, J. and Glasper, E.A. (2007) What impact has NHS reforms had on the provision of children's services in England? The views of senior UK children's nurses. *Journal of Children's and Young People's Nursing*, **1** (1), 341–347. You should be able to download a full copy free of charge. Use your highlighter pens to help you follow the process.

The advantage of any critique framework is that it provides structure to your thinking and helps you get some depth to your analysis of an article. It will provide some trigger points that will help you give a balanced view of the article, which is the aim of critiquing, as it should allow you to balance both strengths

---

How to Write Your Nursing Dissertation, First Edition. Alan Glasper and Colin Rees.
© 2013 John Wiley & Sons, Ltd. Published 2013 by John Wiley & Sons, Ltd.

and any limitations to studies. In your dissertation, it is important to say which framework you have used and to indicate any particular reason for your choice.

Although you should use a structured approach on each article, when you include a study in your dissertation you will not write in such depth covering all the points in the framework for each article. The idea is for you to get to the heart of the article and then later decide if you will combine it with other authors making the same point or whether you will highlight key aspects of it that will support your dissertation aim. You will see in Sam's critique that he has made use of the research texts to provide evidence that he understands the issues he has highlighted. He has not simply summarised the article, as that is not the nature of a critique, but has tried to illustrate his understanding of the research elements in the study. Including these kinds of 'explanation' statements in your dissertation can help gain marks.

Here is Sam's critique as it might appear in his dissertation notes using each of the headings in the Rees framework.

Article: Ellis J and Glasper EA (2007) What impact has NHS reforms had on the provision of children's services in England? The views of senior UK children's nurses.

1   Focus

The focus of this article is the impact of government health policy on the delivery of services, and specifically children's health services. The NHS reforms are those of the Labour government up to 2007, which is when the article was published. This is a worthwhile topic for investigation, as it provides an assessment of the impact of policy on clinical practice and the delivery of care in a specialist clinical area.

2   Background

The background to the study is set within the context of health policy reforms and the way in which these affected the structure of healthcare in England, specifically in children's services leading up to 2007. The trigger for the study was an approach by the Department of Health (in England) to the Association of Chief Children's Nurses (ACCN) to set up a study to find out the answer to this question of policy impact. Unusually for a research study, there is no clear review of the literature section examining current research knowledge on the topic. There is a short summary in the introduction that suggests there are negative views on the effectiveness of the new policies that affect children's services. None of the sources included in the section are research studies. The inclusion of this literature provides some justification for carrying out the present study. A review of the literature including research studies would have enabled the reader to place the topic within the context of current evidence and research on the topic. It must be presumed that no such studies have been completed and this study may be breaking new ground.

3 **Aim**

There is no subheading or statement regarding the aim of the study. However, the aim can be identified both in the abstract and early in the introduction in identical words as part of the explanation for the way the study was developed. The aim appears to be 'to consider what impact NHS reforms have had on the provision of children's services in England'. The statement of the aim is important in any study as Lacey (2010) has pointed out that it will influence the type of research approach needed to answer it. In this study, the statement of the aim does not indicate the sample from which the data will be collected, which often forms part of such statements. However, from the title of the article, the sample related to the aim is 'senior UK children's nurses'. There is a single variable in the aim which is 'impact of the NHS reforms on children's services' that suggests that the most appropriate method would be a descriptive survey. This, according to Burns and Grove (2009), is a really useful way of collecting data from a group of people.

4 **Study design**

This takes a quantitative design where the numbers of those agreeing to a list of statements is sought through a questionnaire-type technique, and the results presented in numeric tables. This is a key feature of quantitative studies that examine numerically features of a variable (Holland and Rees, 2010). A quantitative approach is appropriate for the research question posed here, which attempts to measure the amount of agreement on an issue, and the tables of numeric results confirm this is the approach used.

5 **Data collection method**

The data collection method was the use a Delphi instrument. This is like a questionnaire but has a series of statements that have been constructed by an 'expert panel' (Tappen, 2011). Here, the list of statements was produced by a focus group of 19 members of the ACCN at one of its meetings. In common with other such studies, there is no mention of a pilot of the questionnaire (Keeney, 2010), which raises the issue of the reliability of the tool, in other words whether or not it is measuring accurately and consistently (Holland and Rees, 2010). Pilot studies also allow the wording of questions to be checked for understanding by those who make up the sample. Respondents show their level of support for each item in the list using a five-point Likert scale. This is one of the most popular attitude scales (Burns and Grove, 2009) where respondents choose a response from 'strongly agree' to 'strongly disagree' for each statement. As the list of the items in the Delphi instrument is included in the article, it is possible to see that only one statement is worded in the positive, the majority have negative wordings attached to them, such as 'stifled', 'burden', 'inadequate', 'inappropriate' and so on. This could lead to a bias in responses, as respondents have only a majority of negative statements from which to make their choice. Controlling bias, or distortion, in a study is important as it affects the accuracy of the results (Rees, 2011). It also raises the issue of validity, specifically, have the researchers measured what they believe they have measured (Polit and Beck, 2008), as respondents may be subconsciously influenced by the negative wording to see the topic in a negative light. This means the results may be more to do with the structure of the data collection tool rather than the respondent's own views.

6 **Ethical considerations**

There is little mention of ethical issues in the article, such as approval by an ethics committee. However, it is important to acknowledge that these were not patients but senior nurses and were representing members of a professional society. The method is not invasive, although Keeney (2010) does point out there can be issues of coercion involved, that is, pressure to take part, and Delphi instruments should be treated like questionnaires when it comes to ethical considerations. The only ethical issue mentioned in the article was anonymity, which was achieved for round two of the questionnaire. The omission of ethical issues is not felt to be a problem here.

7 **Sample**

Sampling can be identified at two points in the study. Firstly, the tool of data collection was designed by an opportunity sample of members of the ACCN who were attending a meeting. Secondly, this tool was then mailed to those on the list of the society asking them to participate in the study. The results are based on returns from 11 members who were on the Association of Chief Children's Nurses (ACCN) list. However, it is not until the conclusion section that we learn this is out of a possible total of 27 participants who are on the list of those still involved in the delivery of children's services. Therefore, this represents a response rate of 40%. This raises questions of who the results represent. Such a small number may not represent the views of this body or, in fact, those working in services for children. There are no stated sample inclusion or exclusion criteria to help in deciding how representative the sample is, as the only inclusion criteria were that respondents had to be on the ACCN group list and decide to return the Delphi questionnaire. Although bias may not be the major issue in this kind of exploratory study, it is difficult to make generalisations from this sample. This sampling approach forms an opportunity or convenience sample, which is one that is easy to access but may be open to bias (Burns and Grove, 2009).

8 **Data presentation**

The principles of quantitative research have been followed here (Holland and Rees, 2010), where most of the results are described in terms of the numbers agreeing with the statements in the Delphi tool. There is only one table of the results that contains statements where at least 70% of the 11 respondents said they agreed or strongly agreed with the statement. This means that the statements were support by between 8 and 11 of the respondents. One criticism of the table is that it would have been easier to read if statements with the same 'score' had been grouped together rather than presented in no particular order. That is, if all the items supported by 11 respondents were grouped first followed by the items supported by 10 and so on. This would then meet the criteria for constructing tables suggested by Burns and Grove (2009) – that tables should allow the reader to easily review the contents.

9 **Main findings**

The main finding from the study is that, in the view of the sample of members of the ACCN group completing this Delphi survey, the NHS reforms are seen in a negative light. There are 20 items that received a 70% level of consensus amongst the 11 members involved in this study, five items were agreed by all 11. One of these, 'Children's commissioning not strong', is highlighted by the authors as one of the major criticisms of the government reforms. However, this is not supported by any other details to help the reader understand why this is more important than the other categories mentioned by all 11 respondents.

10 **Conclusion and recommendations**

It is disappointing to find that there is not a clear conclusion or any recommendations to this study. The nearest to a conclusion is listed in the table of 'key points', where it is stated: 'Some NHS reforms have had a negative impact on the delivery of children's services in English hospitals' (Ellis and Glasper, 2007). This is supported by some of the items in the list of the data collection tool. However, we must remember that the statements are more personal opinions and are not supported by any service outcome data. Nearly all the items were expressed using negative wording, so this conclusion is not surprising. In relation to 'where do we go from here', which is the purpose of recommendations, there are no suggestions for what might improve the situation (Rees, 2011).

11 **Readability**

The article covers the 'bigger picture' of health policy and NHS reforms. As such, the emphasis is on service structure and delivery. This topic may not be of interest to everyone. On the whole the language is simple. The methodological sections are quite brief. There is a clear and informative description of the Delphi technique. In the results sections, the items in the tool of data collection are discussed in some depth, unusually for a results section, these are supported by comments from the literature. Some elements, such as how many people were in the ACCN focus group, were difficult to find, as they were not always in the place they are usually located in a research article. The lack of a clear conclusion and recommendations was surprising, as it gave the article a feeling of being incomplete.

12   Practice implications

The main practice implications relate to the realisation from this study that there are a number of pressures in the clinical area that are the result of policy changes. The study identifies that government reforms, rather than improving the situation, can make practice more of a challenge, at least from the perspective of senior nurses. Although it was interesting to read about a research technique that can be easily used to gain a consensus view from a group, the study has not added a great deal to our knowledge on the impact of NHS reforms on children's services in England, other than suggesting they were unpopular with a group of senior nurses. This may require a different form of study, such as a larger survey of clinical staff, and a quantification of some outcome measures and service delivery figures to provide greater understanding.

Conclusion

This model for critiquing has allowed Sam to approach quite a difficult article in a systematic way by concentrating on the structure and quality of the research element. You will notice that Sam has tried to go further than simply describing each element such as 'they used such-and-such tool' or 'there were so many people in the study'. Instead, he has tried to consider the implications of the points raised and tries to help the reader assess the quality of the study through his evaluations. He has also followed academic convention and avoided the use of 'I think' to express his views. It is still clear, however, that the views are his and he has not simply summarised the article but critically evaluated it.

A point made at the start of this section was that Sam has made use of the research text books to support his comments. At degree and master's level, part of successful academic writing is illustrating that you understand issues and can support your statements by drawing on the work of experts in that topic area. Sam has wisely used more than one research text book to show that he has read around the topic of research and can use this to underpin his arguments, using a very natural and informative style of writing.

References

Burns, N. and Grove, S. (2009) *The Practice of Nursing Research: Appraisal, Synthesis, and Generation of Evidence* (6th edn). Saunders, St Louis.

Ellis, J. and Glasper, E.A. (2007) What impact has NHS reforms had on the provision of children's services in England? The views of senior UK children's nurses. *Journal of Children's and Young People's Nursing*, **1** (1), 341–347.

Holland, K. and Rees, C. (2010) *Nursing: Evidence-Based Practice Skills*. Oxford University Press, Oxford.

Keeney, S. (2010) The Delphi Technique. In: K. Gerrish and A. Lacey (eds), The Research Process in Nursing (6th edn). Chichester: Wiley-Blackwell.

Lacey, A. (2010) The research process. In: A Gerrish and A Lacey (eds.) *The Research Process in Nursing* (6th edn). John Wiley & Sons Ltd, Chichester.

Polit, D. and Beck, C. (2008) *Nursing Research: Generating and Assessing Evidence for Nursing Practice* (8th edn). Lippincott Williams and Wilkins, Philadelphia, PA.

Rees, C. (2011) *Introduction to Research for Midwives* (3rd edn). Churchill Livingstone, Edinburgh.

Tappen, R. (2011) *Advanced Nursing Research: From Theory to Practice*. Jones and Bartlett Learning, Sudbury.

For further resources for this chapter visit the companion website at

   www.wiley.com/go/glasper/nursingdissertation

Section 6 **How evidence-based healthcare is implemented in practice**

Over coffee Sam tells Sue that he has a great lead for his dissertation. He has found a range of papers on work done in Sydney Children's Hospital, where they have had success in implementing evidence-based practice. Additionally, Sue has read some of Professor Peter Callery's work.

Chapter 20   **Using evidence in practice**

Tracey Harding[1], Lisa Harding[2] and Alan Glasper[1]
[1]*University of Southampton, UK*
[2]*University of Winchester, UK*

> **Scenario**
>
> Sue is writing the final chapter of her dissertation and has to consider how evidence is embedded in practice. She has been advised to consider all aspects of the change process.

Introduction

This chapter explores how evidence can be shared with practice colleagues and the wider audience. It also explains why it is important to share knowledge and change practice as a result of evidence that has been critiqued and assessed for its credibility and applicability. Leadership and change management theory will be explored in relation to implementing change in practice. The global dissemination of nursing knowledge comes about through reading peer reviewed publications and an understanding of research findings and their implications for practice. Harnessing change management theory for the purposes of changing practice, based on best evidence, remains challenging and is often the subject of a separate chapter for dissertation students undertaking an evidence-based practice project as part of a degree pathway.

This chapter will continue Sue's dissertation journey. She has now critiqued relevant literature, assessing it for its validity and applicability to her own area of investigation; she feels now that she would like to implement the findings in the form of change within her ward. Sam's experience is that many students, once they have completed their dissertation, rarely proceed to local implementation of their findings in practice, so he is encouraging Sue to consider local implementation with a view to going beyond this and continue sharing what she has learnt and encourage implementation of the findings to a wider audience.

How to Write Your Nursing Dissertation, First Edition. Alan Glasper and Colin Rees.
© 2013 John Wiley & Sons, Ltd. Published 2013 by John Wiley & Sons, Ltd.

Scenario

Sue's project for her dissertation has explored the importance of rest for patients whilst in hospital recovering from illness and following a critique of relevant literature wants to implement findings in her practice. Sue wants to propose that a dedicated time is allocated as a 'rest period' for patients where lighting can be reduced, effort made by all staff to keep noise levels to a minimum, visiting is restricted to outside of the rest period and where, additionally, multiprofessional care/treatment interventions can be scheduled outside of this time. Sue and Sam regularly meet for coffee; Sue discusses with Sam a starting point for her plans for implementation. Many staff working on her ward have been aware of Sue's dissertation topic and have been kept up to date with the findings from the literature Sue has critiqued. However, Sue now needs to implement the change within her practice setting. The ward sister is reluctant to make the change Sue wants to implement, arguing 'things are just fine the way they are'.

The ward sister feels it would be difficult to change the way people work and outlines some of the difficulties she foresees – '*What about the doctors rounds, are we just going to ask them not to come during the rest period? And physiotherapists, are we supposed to ask them not to get patients out of bed during this stated period? I can't see them agreeing to that*'.

Sue now feels a bit demotivated and seeks advice from Sam.

Applying research findings to practice: using and applying evidence in practice

The global dissemination of nursing knowledge continues to be debated. However, it is agreed that the dissemination of ideas through and within disciplines can be developed as a result of peer reviewed publications, where knowledge is developed and challenged (Holt *et al.*, 2000). Change is an essential component of nursing practice, where translation of research findings into practice may increase the effectiveness of patient care (Nemeth, 2003). It is acknowledged that throughout healthcare, there is an interest in promoting evidence-based practice. However, despite a vision within the healthcare professions to integrate research findings into practice, how this happens in reality is given limited consideration (Stetler, 2003). Leeman *et al.* (2007) highlight that over the last two decades more effective methods to promote the use of best practice by both clinicians and healthcare organisations have been sought. McGlynn *et al.* (2003) and Hussey *et al.* (2004) argue that the gap between what is known to be best practice with what care patients receive, continues to grow wider.

It is understood that from both professional and economic perspectives, care given within the NHS needs to be determined by the best available evidence (Alfaro-LeFevre, 2004). The implementation of best practice is recognised as incredibly complex, being dependent on people and the multiple influences that are involved (Greenhalgh, 2006). In July 2010, as a prelude to the NHS White Paper *Equality and Excellence: Liberating the NHS* (DH, 2010a), the Chief Nursing Officer for England published *High Impact Actions for Nursing and Midwifery: The Essential Collection*, which presented eight case studies taken from practice to illustrate potential savings of millions within the NHS. These examples illustrate practice innovation aiming to improve the quality of patient care whilst demonstrating reduction in costs (Glasper, 2010a).

Scenario

During an afternoon shift Sue and Sam meet during their break. They begin discussing the importance of using evidence in practice.

Having still only written chapter two in draft form, the chapter where it relates to the search for literature, Sue has included some references regarding what evidence-based practice is and feels this needs emphasising throughout the project.

Sam agrees, reinforcing to Sue that as she is aiming to review her practice and that of others, to search for evidence related to a specific area, critically assess the evidence for its applicability and explore whether it answers her project question; the aim being to improve practice. Sam continues by adding that nurses need to explore evidence to ensure the best care possible is provided (Burns and Grove, 2009) which of course can help with decision making (Sackett *et al.*, 1996; Greenhalgh, 2006). Sam is adamant that patients are included in the decisions about their care and argues that nurses need to be able to inform patients of the options.

Sue thinks about this for a minute and begins to realise that it is more than just knowing about one type of treatment option and their likely outcomes; nurses need to be aware of other options and help the patient to make the right decision for them. Furthermore, she realises that it is also important to be aware that practitioners do not and will not know all the best practices supported by research, so the importance of sharing knowledge is ever more crucial.

Sam tells Sue about an article he has read recently that had discussed best practice and the environment in which this could be cultivated. It had argued that the organisational culture needed to foster an environment where care is based on best available research that has been skilfully and knowledgeably interpreted, through the judgements of clinically competent practitioners, combined with patient desires to develop quality outcomes (Fineout-Overholt and Melnyk, 2005). After giving further thought to this, Sam suggested that when people talk about 'best practice' it does not just mean within healthcare, it refers to other business organisations too, so the culture in any organisation is important, it needs to be collaborative, value driven and involve the sharing of successful solutions (Fineout-Overholt and Melnyk, 2005).

Sam suggests that Sue thinks about the terms 'dissemination' of research and 'implementation' for a minute, and asks her to consider the differences. Sue thinks about this and proposes that dissemination is sharing ideas and implementation is putting the ideas into practice. Sam once again agrees; dissemination involves the promotion of research messages and the implementation involves getting the findings of research used in practice (NHS Centre for Reviews and Dissemination, 1999). There may not be any point in undertaking research if you have no intention of sharing the findings with practitioners, because essential to the whole research process is the dissemination of new knowledge and, of course, changing behaviour (Dunn *et al.*, 1994; Crosswaite and Curtice, 1994).

Sue expresses concern regarding the implementation of the project findings in her practice environment; she is aware of the high turnover of staff and is worried this may affect implementation. The ward sister has recently informed ward staff during morning report that there will be more staff changes in the next week or so; two members of staff are leaving, one due to retirement and one to a nearby ward. Sam highlights to Sue that high levels of staff turnover are quite common to unstable environments and, if continuing, may affect commitment to the change (Buckwalter *et al.*, 2009). Sam makes reference to his experiences over the years as a practitioner within the National Health Service (NHS), commenting that there may also be opposing attitudes, entrenched practices and habitual service delivery that impede the achievement of goals (Lacey, 1994). All of which, Sam continues, need to be considered when planning any new initiatives.

Greenhalgh (2006) recognises that, generally, an organisation will adopt new practices more willingly if the practice is well established, if resources, for example, money and staffing, are minimal and where teams can work autonomously. Furthermore, it is recognised that research compatible with current government thinking or which is timely is more likely to be used (Thomas, 1985). However, whatever theoretical approach is taken to implement a change in practice, it is recognised that the challenge will be tough.

Evidence exists in many forms and the term 'level of evidence' often relates to the study design and nature of the article, with systematic reviews of randomised controlled trials being considered the best form of evidence

(Greenhalgh, 2006). However, the research design needs to be taken into consideration in relation to the research question, so therefore needs to be relevant. Effective healthcare strategies often take some time, years even, to catch on. The reason for this is thought to be because the implementation of best practice is highly complex, involving numerous influences and is dependent on people with their individual personalities and the effect they can have on each other and also the context of the environment (Greenhalgh, 2006).

So local implementation would seem to be the *first step*, but evaluation of its implementation and audit of its success are necessary to establish commitment and effect of the change. However, consideration also needs to be given to sharing research findings to a wider audience.

The way research is presented and communicated can influence whether it is used (Parahoo, 2006) AND if communicated in a language that practitioners understand, publication in scientific journals is a suitable forum of exchange of information (Cullum, 2000; Oermann *et al.*, 2008). To ensure that the findings/outcomes of local implementation from Sue's dissertation reach relevant practitioners it is advised that findings should be published in clinical journals, where they should be easy to read and the implications for practice are emphasised (Veeramah, 2004) (Chapter 21, Publishing your dissertation: in a journal or at a conference).

It is important to stress that nurses and others need knowledge of and about research to make use of findings. Therefore, education is a necessary condition for integrating research and practice, though not the only prerequisite, as the context in which the implementation takes place is important (Parahoo, 1997).

Kitson *et al.* (1998) have suggested that the implementation of change to practice is most successful when the evidence is robust, the context is receptive to the change and the process of change is facilitated appropriately. McCormack *et al.* (2002) explored the concept of 'context' in relation to successful implementation of evidence in practice, and found that the term 'context' is inconsistently used. McCormack *et al.* (2002) suggest that, in relation to the complexity of healthcare environments, 'context' implies more than simply the environment and the culture of that environment, and should include, as equally important factors, 'systems of decision making, staff relationships, organisational systems, power differentials and the potential of the organisation to innovate' (p. 101).

To ensure a successful transfer of knowledge into practice, it is recommended that a variety of dissemination strategies is used, that they are supported by organisational incentives and involve researchers, practitioners, and policy makers (Dunn *et al.*, 1994). Communication in professions such as nursing shares a category of knowledge in common with other disciplines, namely interaction (Sheldon and Ellington, 2008) and is, therefore, deemed critical during the implementation phase of any change (Allen *et al.*, 2007; Lines, 2004).

It is recognised that both leadership and decision making can influence healthcare provision positively, if implemented effectively (Harding and Sque, 2010). Healthcare professionals have experienced an increasing emphasis on their ability to account for decisions they make and with greater transparency (Thompson and Dowding, 2002) and with a need to behave in a consciously political way in relation to decision making, as opposed to simply replying on the position of professional expert (Young and Cooke, 2002). Researchers continue to seek better ways to make decisions and the ability to make a wise proactive decision is of benefit for any leader within healthcare and at any level (Wheeler, 2000, cited in Bower, 2000, p. 199). It has been mentioned earlier that exploring and using evidence in practice can aid decision making. This section provides justification for this and demonstrates how evidence-based practice can influence critical thinking and decision making.

The developing culture within healthcare practice is one that is moving away from delivering care according to tradition, towards making use of research and evidence (Tod *et al.*, 2004), challenging healthcare professionals to justify decisions made, basing them on best available evidence (Pinch, 2001). It is important to acknowledge that evidence may not provide absolute certainty and practice recommendations may change as new research emerges (Rycroft-Malone *et al.*, 2004).

Sam advises Sue, therefore, that it is essential to develop increasing research awareness with a continuous review of practices, as the research evidence for practice is constantly evolving.

A distinction has been made between problem solving and decision making. Higgins (1991) argues that in problem solving, the issue is whether the decision made was a good one; according to whether the problem is solved, and Wheeler (2000, cited in Bower, 2000, p199) states that this differs to decision making, where there is a choice to be made, following consideration of alternatives, therefore one makes choices from a variety of options, meaning that decision making may not necessarily include a problem, and may or may not create a favourable outcome.

Sam sees Sue in the staff restaurant, he sits beside her and they catch up on her progress with her dissertation. Sue tells Sam she is exploring how evidence is used in decision making. Sam asks Sue to imagine that she is looking after a patient, that her knowledge of the condition which attributed to the patients hospital admission was limited, that the patient's condition deteriorated and that she was required to take action. It is recognised that often associated with accuracy is experience (Gordon, 1980; Thompson and Dowding, 2002). Healthcare knowledge has been influenced by other disciplines, such as psychology, sociology and anatomy and physiology, and although this informs practice it does not constitute healthcare knowledge (Berragan, 1998). Sam talks about the 'practice' of nursing as being something more than the description offered above and asks Sue if she has heard of Carper, a name often spoken of in relation to nursing knowledge. Sam continues to describe Carper's (1978) fundamental patterns of knowing in nursing. There are four ways of knowing: empirical, the science of nursing; ethical, the component of moral knowledge; aesthetic, the art of nursing, perception, understanding and intuition; and personal knowledge in nursing. Sam and Sue explore care given to a specific patient that morning and identify how and what knowledge they drew upon to inform their decision making. Sue soon realised she had been able to draw upon her own experiences in practice and knowledge from her nurse training and that which followed after qualifying, which had been judged credible. In addition to this, Sue had sought the experiences of Sam, an expert in his field of practice.

Arbon (2004) argues that knowledge that underpins expert nursing in practice is accumulative and is derived from learning about practice in real and often complex situations. Once again, however, Sam proposes that this is not as straightforward as it sounds.

Arbon (2004:152) continues to argue that nursing expertise and how nurses practise is more complex, stating that for many nurses, 'experience generates meanings and understandings about themselves and others that appear to be individual, personal and transferable across fields of practice'. Sue furthermore realised that the patient, too, offered insight into the decision to be made, where jointly a way forward and treatment options had been agreed.

> Using knowledge and experience may help to predict events, and therefore steps may then be taken to avoid deterioration or at least enable a position to manage it, be prepared for it.

Bower (2000) argues that being proactive in decision making involves having the ability to anticipate the event. There needs to be consideration of the choice to be selected, in addition to the consideration of the context of that decision and how it may affect the outcome of the decision. It could be argued that being in a position to do this means having an awareness of practice which is informed by evidence. Wheeler (2000, cited in Bower, 2000, p. 206) confirms that 'being proactive involves keeping abreast of new techniques and theories for improving the workplace' and is supported by Thompson and Dowding (2002:3) who state that good decisions are born by virtue of 'clinical expertise and knowledge generated by good quality research'. However, Berragan (1998) argues that not all clinical situations have a scientific answer, thus sources of knowledge should not be judged against each other but given value for their own purpose. Redelmeier *et al.* (2001) advise that clinical judgement combines scientific theory, personal experience and patient perspectives.

Nursing has developed into the realms of diagnosis, screening patient and providing prognosis (Thompson and Dowding, 2002) where Hedberg and Satterlund Larsson (2003) recognise that nurse's decision making in clinical practice uses two knowledge domains, that of nursing and medicine. From the medical perspective, the decisions nurses make are based on delegated responsibility, based on their assessment of the patient, often informed by evidence-based guidelines and descriptive directives relating to procedures for example Nurses and other healthcare professionals are often involved in complex situations and decisions that need in-depth thinking. Alfaro-LeFevre (2004) argues there is a difference between thinking and critical thinking, saying that critical thinking is purposeful and controlled and focuses on well-reasoned strategies, where new ideas may be developed and analysed.

It is acknowledged that perhaps during times of high pressure within care delivery there is a tendency to undertake care which is based on tradition rather than research. However, asking questions about care, asking how and why practices are undertaken, encourages critical thinking of guidelines (Alfaro-LeFevre, 2004) and with access to research literature enables up-to-date and credible findings to be explored.

Ethical considerations are associated with decision making and the outcomes of care maybe of interest from personal, financial and social perspectives, where service users have greater influence in their own treatment and the way the NHS operates (Young and Cooke, 2002). Sue was able to appreciate this, when reflecting on a decision made earlier that day. Later when together with Sam they explored their use of knowledge to inform their decision making.

Scenario

Sam and Sue consider the journey they have taken with regard to discussions about Sue's project. They think about the context of Sue's ward initiative, how it may affect the use of resources, how it affects patients/service users and their relatives, what the benefits might be, the impact on teamwork/multiprofessional working, and any ethical implications and political influences that may be apparent. Evidence can inform/aid decision making and the natural sciences continue to provide health workers with useful information upon which clinical judgement is based (Berragan, 1998).

Sue and Sam discuss the timeliness of changing practice and how creative an initiative might be. Sam suggests that creativity in clinical practice has its place, arguing that it needs to consider many factors, including the assessment of ideas to ensure usefulness to the end user. This is where exploring the evidence is essential; thought needs to be given to what research is saying in relation to ideas and how it can be applied to get the best results.

Potential barriers to the implementation of change

This section explores and includes a discussion of how to implement findings into practice, giving consideration to the culture of the organisation, leadership styles and change management strategies best suited to achieve this.

Impediments to change

Following her conversation with Sam, Sue takes some time to reflect on the discussion and consider some of the impediments to implementing the changes on a local basis. In considering these potential impediments, Sue is hoping that she can find ways of reducing or eliminating them in order to ensure the successful implementation of the change initiative, in relation to provision of dedicated time allocated as a 'rest period' for patients.

Sue recalls that her discussion with Sam highlighted the following:

- The ward sister is reluctant to implement changes, as she is concerned how other members of the multiprofessional team will react to the restrictions that these changes may impose on their ability to fulfil their activities, for example, doctor's rounds.
- There is already a high turnover of staff on the ward and the ward sister has recently informed staff that there will be more staff changes in the near future as two further members of staff are leaving. Whilst recognising that high staff turnover is quite common in unstable environments, Sue knows that if this situation persists this may affect staff commitment to the change (Buckwalter *et al.*, 2009).

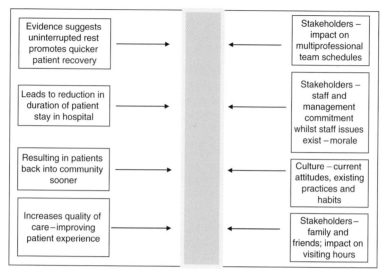

Figure 20.1   Lewin's Force Field Analysis: an example

- Sam has advised that opposing attitudes, entrenched practices and habitual service delivery can impede the achievement of goals (Lacey, 1994) and that these need to be considered when planning any new initiatives.

Sue realises that these could potentially be significant impediments to the successful implementation of her change initiative and decides to investigate further the implications of these, and other potential impediments that she is likely to encounter, when seeking to implement 'rest periods' for patients.

Sue decides to use Lewin's Force Field Analysis to help identify the 'drivers' and 'resistors' to change (Rollinson, 2008; Cameron and Green, 2009; Nelson and Quick 2011) (Figure 20.1). Additionally Lewin's change management model, which will be discussed later, is very helpful in understanding how to implements change, and his concept of unfreezing the current situation and then changing the situation before finally refreezing into the new service delivery model has stood the test of time The change management model, which is this three-stage process, is analogous to changing the shape of ice, so to make a ball of ice into a cube first requires unfreezing, then reshaping before finally refreezing.

Stakeholder resistance

Employee resistance to change falls into four broad categories: parochial self-interest, misunderstanding, a different perspective or assessment of the current situation and low tolerance to change (Bedeian and Zammuto, 1991, cited in Rollinson, 2008, p. 639).

> **Summary table**
>
> *In summary when considering impediments to change:*
> - *Using Lewin's Force Field Analysis and management change model can help to identify drivers – forces for change and forces resisting change.*
> - *In the analysis consider all stakeholders, for example, management, staff, customers (patients, family and friends), suppliers, partners (multiprofessional team) and community as appropriate.*
> - *Other factors to take into consideration include the culture of the organisation/ department/team and how that might affect successful implementation of change as well as any relevant internal and external factors, such as budget and legislation/regulation.*

Employees are only interested in how change impacts on them as individuals and their future rather than the success of the organisation. Misunderstanding can arise as a result of inadequate or untimely information, which may diminish trust and could result in employees seeking an alternative explanation as to why changes are being introduced. This could lead to resistance to, or sabotage of, change. In addition, there may be some individuals who are fearful of a new process which may undermine their self-belief. Therefore, habit and loss of freedom, security in the past and fear of the unknown can be contributors to resistance (Robbins, 2001; Mullins, 2010).

In addition, group inertia, threats to power, expertise and resources may increase resistance to change (Robbins, 2001; Rollinson, 2008; Mullins, 2010). Groups and teams develop their own patterns of behaviour (norms) which may be threatened by change. In the same way, change may be perceived to be reducing responsibility and freedom in decision making. In this case, this may apply to the multiprofessional team and the ward manager. Indeed, management has been identified as being the biggest barrier to change, innovation and new ideas (Teal, 1998).

Consequently, Sue realises that when considering implementing change it is important for individuals and teams to:

- Understand how changes impact them individually and their future. If they believe they are losing something they value, they will resist, and may collaborate to block change.
- Believe the rationale for change as good enough for change to be implemented, otherwise they may make alternative conclusions which could lead to resistance.

As the agent for change, it is important for Sue to understand that individuals value security and stability in their work, and therefore the introduction of a new process may undermine their self-belief. It is important that fear of change is recognised and reassurance provided, otherwise individuals and teams may resist change. Information should be adequate, timely and communicated effectively and Sue needs to understand that, even with open consultation, it is important not to assume, that resistance may exist. Communication has a key role to play in this process as change is implemented and sustained through communication (Russ, 2008). This is supported by Kotter *et al.* (1986 cited in Rollinson, 2008, p. 640) who suggest there are seven ways of reducing resistance to change: education and communication, participation, facilitation and support, negotiation and, when the situation requires, co-optation, manipulation and coercion.

Sue concludes that as a result of her investigation the needs of other stakeholders, including the multiprofessional team, family and friends and any other function/department affected by the introduction of 'rest periods', need to be considered during the implementation stage. Ways in which they can be consulted and informed of any plans, with details of how the change will affect them, the benefits of the change and opportunities for them to ask questions and provide feedback need to be included.

Summary Table

In summary when seeking to reduce/eliminate resistance to change it is important to:
- *Ensure the rationale for the change is communicated.*
- *Ensure the changes are communicated in terms of the benefits to the individual as well as, in this case, the patient and the organisation.*
- *Ensure information provided is adequate and timely to avoid misunderstandings.*
- *Recognise that fear of change may exist and provide reassurance.*
- *Recognise that effective communication is required <u>throughout</u> the process.*
- *Encourage participation of others in the change process.*

Organisational culture

The way in which individuals undertake their roles is what creates and maintains the culture of an organisation (Wilson, 1992). Many definitions of organisational culture exist, where it is thought that the culture provides shared meanings, obligations, understanding and expectations (Anthony, 1994). The culture therefore influences values and behaviours of its workforce (Young and Cooke, 2002).

It is important to understand the extent to which culture can be changed and how the changes can be made, as 'the enthusiasts who unwittingly work counter-culturally will find that there is a metaphorical but solid brick wall against which they are beating their heads' (Torrington *et al.*, 2002:96–97). The culture required for successful implementation of change is one of collaboration, one that is value driven and involves the sharing of successful solutions (Fineout-Overholt and Melnyk, 2005).

Summary Table

In summary, when implementing change think about how the culture of the organisation or department might affect the change process, for example:
- *Is the culture one that will readily accept and embrace change?*
- *How does the planned change 'fit' with practices and customs already in place?*
- *How much does the existing culture value, for example, collaboration?*
- *Who are the key players in this culture?*

Sue now has a 'checklist' for the implementation of her change initiative. This, Sue believes, will help her to evaluate different change management strategies for use in the implementing the planned changes.

Change management strategies

Some change management processes suggest that change is a rational, ordered process that can be controlled when, in practice, it can be chaotic involving surprising events and unexpected outcomes (Anderson, 2002:339). Some experiences of implementation of evidence in practice indicate it is messy and presents challenges which are not easily represented by rational models (Rycroft-Malone *et al.*, 2002). It is suggested that successful implementation of change is dependent upon the quality of implementation, the consideration given to other stakeholder perspectives and the level of support provided by those with influence in the organisation, as well as the change approach adopted (Anderson, 2002:340). With this in mind, Sue investigates and evaluates several change management strategies for use in implementing her change initiative.
- Lewin – Three-Step Model

The term 'planned change' was first introduced by Kurt Lewin to indicate change that is consciously planned by an organisation rather than change that occurs by accident or that is forced upon the organisation (Burnes, 2000). Lewin suggests that in order to be successful, change should involve movement through three stages: *unfreezing* of the present state, *movement* to the new state and *refreezing* of the new state. The model places emphasis on the importance of 'felt-need' and activities undertaken within the unfreezing and movement stages should convince stakeholders of the need for change. Links between these two stages of Lewin's (1951) model and Action Research have been made, where unfreezing relates to the research element and movement relates to the action element (Burnes, 2000). A summary of the three-step model is detailed in Figure 20.2.

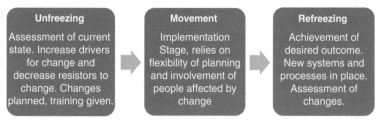

Unfreezing	Movement	Refreezing
Assessment of current state. Increase drivers for change and decrease resistors to change. Changes planned, training given.	Implementation Stage, relies on flexibility of planning and involvement of people affected by change	Achievement of desired outcome. New systems and processes in place. Assessment of changes.

Figure 20.2   Lewin's three-step model

Sue, using this model, maps out how she might approach the implementation of her change initiative (Table 20.1).

The three steps in this model are broad and have been subsequently further developed to provide practical value to implementation of change (Burnes, 2000). The model, whilst acknowledging the importance of 'felt need' and of decreasing resistors to change, does not sufficiently highlight the importance of the energy of the key players in the change process (Cameron and Green, 2009). Sue, therefore, decides to investigate further models which not only take into consideration 'felt-need' but also consider key players in the change process.

- Bullock and Batten (1985) – Planned Change

This model describes planned change in terms of four change phases and their change processes (Cameron and Green, 2009), as illustrated in Figure 20.3.

Whilst this model has applicability to many organisations (Cummings and Huse, 1989, cited in Burnes, 2000, p. 272) it assumes that change can be defined, and achieved, in a planned approach. It assumes that organisational change is a technical problem and, therefore, solved with a technical solution (Cameron and Green, 2009). In assessing this model, Sue also acknowledges that whilst this it is useful for approaching less complex change initiatives, it ignores any potential resistance to change and does not take into account the interdependencies between the different business units – for example, in this case the ward and the multiprofessional team.

- PDSA Cycle

The PDSA cycle cited by le May in Chapter 4 (What is evidence-based practice and clinical effectiveness) is facilitated through the posing of three specific questions, which includes:

- What is it that the healthcare team is trying to accomplish? When setting goals to achieve the planned change, teams need to use objectives which are specific, measurable, achievable, realistic and time bound (SMART).
- How will the team know that any change they make is an improvement over the previous model? This stage in the PDSA cycle is all about measurement. The essential collection gives 'seven steps to measurement' which seek to measure the effectiveness of any change to patient care or practice.

Table 20.1 Breakdown of Lewin's Three-Step Model

Stage in model	Action	Example
UNFREEZING	What is the current state?	• No 'rest periods' currently on ward • Patients are interrupted regularly • Investigations can be arranged at any time of the day • Patient feedback has intimated that this is frustrating • Research suggests that 'rest periods' facilitate quicker recovery
	What are the driving forces for change and what are the forces for resistance to change?	• Improved quality of care • Improved patient experience • Management resistance to change • High staff turnover • Disruption to multiprofessional team schedules • Impact on visiting hours
	How can change be implemented?	• Explain research to stakeholders, via meetings • Consult manager and staff regarding time for 'rest period' • Create notices for ward and letters for relatives advising of changes
	What training is required Who needs to be communicated with in respect of changes planned?	• No training currently required • Manager • Staff • Multiprofessional team • Relatives • Other hospital staff involved in ward administration and management
MOVEMENT	How can stakeholders be involved in the process?	• Consult and involve stakeholders, such as staff, with regard to introduction of change – it's timing, how to communicate with other stakeholders, how to manage the process
	What flexibility needs to be built into the plan?	• Timing of introduction – for example, staff changes planned in next few weeks • Exceptions to 'rest period', for example, terminally ill, palliative care patients.
REFREEZING	How can changes be reviewed, measured and evaluated?	• Staff and team feedback via discussion and meetings regarding disruption to schedules, workloads and communication • Patient feedback via discussion and surveys regarding quality if care and patient experience • Monitoring length of hospital stay and comparing data to current statistics • Observations of 'rest periods' and feedback
	How can the new process be embedded into practice?	• Formal procedures written and circulated

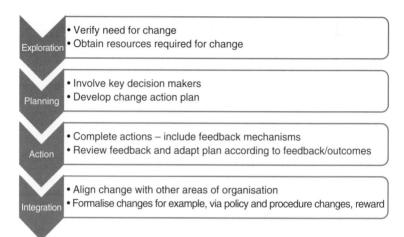

Figure 20.3   Bullock and Batten's (1985) planned change

For further details are given later in this chapter (in the section, Developing a model for improvement).

- Kotter (1995) – Eight-Step Model

This model emphasises the role of the change agent and leadership of the change, and perceives the stages as a process rather than a checklist (Burnes, 2000) (Figure 20.4).

Emergent approaches to change, such as this model, have been criticised for a lack of coherence and validity. However, this approach does suggest that managers should act as facilitators of change and should create a climate that is able to sustain the change by empowering individuals to take responsibility through learning and experimentation (Burnes, 2000). A particular criticism of this model is that the 'energy' levels seem to be high during stages 1–5 and reduce in stages 6–8, whereas the whole process of implementing and sustaining change is challenging and energy needs to be maintained throughout all stages (Cameron and Green, 2009).

Review and evaluation of effectiveness of change

Information collated during implementation, for example staff and patient feedback, can be used to help inform a review of the change. It is important to remember when setting measures for review and evaluation of the change that each stakeholder will hold a different view of the change, have different desired outcomes and, therefore, will perceive success differently (Anderson, 2002:340). These objectives need to be agreed at the outset and Sue is eager to involve as many stakeholders in this process as possible. She suggests to Sam that in

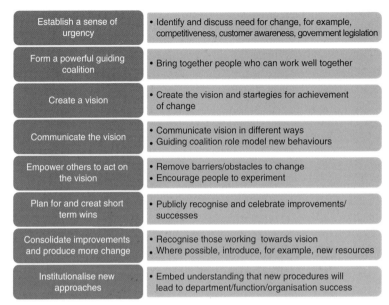

Establish a sense of urgency	• Identify and discuss need for change, for example, competitiveness, customer awareness, government legislation
Form a powerful guiding coalition	• Bring together people who can work well together
Create a vision	• Create the vision and startegies for achievement of change
Communicate the vision	• Communicate vision in different ways • Guiding coalition role model new behaviours
Empower others to act on the vision	• Remove barriers/obstacles to change • Encourage people to experiment
Plan for and creat short term wins	• Publicly recognise and celebrate improvements/successes
Consolidate improvements and produce more change	• Recognise those working towards vision • Where possible, introduce, for example, new resources
Institutionalise new approaches	• Embed understanding that new procedures will lead to department/function/organisation success

Figure 20.4   Kotter's eight-step model (Adapted from Cameron and Green, 2009:115)

Summary Table

In summary when considering how to implement change it is important to remember that change is not always a rational, ordered process and is, in reality, often messy and chaotic. Therefore, it is important to consider:

- *The <u>resources</u> required by the proposed change – are systems, structure, skills and leadership appropriate?*
- *The <u>key players</u> – who are they? How can they be influenced and persuaded that the changes are required? How can their commitment to the change be obtained? To what extent can they be involved in the change process?*
- *The <u>vision</u> – how can the 'vision' for the change be communicated effectively? How can stakeholders be convinced of the rationale for change?*
- *The implementation – what are the <u>SMART objectives</u> for the change? What are the desired outcomes/critical success factors? How can these be achieved? How can the stakeholders be involved? How can feedback be obtained?*
- *The <u>assessment</u> – how will outcomes be measured? How will implementation be reviewed, monitored and evaluated?*
- *<u>Formalising changes</u> – How can changes be embedded to become part of existing practice? Is a formal change in policy/procedure required? If so, who needs to be consulted and/or advised?*

---

her approach she will be looking to reduce the resistors to change by creating a 'vision' of the future in terms of benefits to all stakeholders, consulting with the managers, staff on the ward and the multiprofessional team. She suggests

---

Scenario

Sue arranges to meet with Sam to discuss her findings and plan her approach to implementing the change initiative. She knows that she has an important role in persuading and influencing stakeholders of the need for change, gaining their commitment to the change and ensuring that the change is sustained in the long term. Sue also knows that it is important to set objectives in order that the effectiveness of the change can be measured and evaluated.

---

that this may be achieved by way of a team meeting, presentations and one-to-one discussions. In addition, Sue is looking to communicate her dissertation findings to the staff on the notice board as her literature review provides evidence to support the initiative. Sue is anxious to ensure that she discusses and agrees with the ward manager, as well as coordinating with the multiprofessional team, ways of recognising, promoting and celebrating successes, such as improvement in patient experience feedback and any reduction in patient stay in hospital, to embed the change initiative.

Sam advises Sue that the NHS Plan (DH, 1999a) identified that the development of leadership throughout the NHS could be a vehicle for taking changes forward and that clinical leadership has been acknowledged as being essential for the development of nursing and healthcare practice (Offredy, 1998; Johns, 2003). This, Sam highlights, is a concept also recognised within two UK government strategy documents, *Vision for the Future* (DH, 1993) and *Making a Difference* (DH, 1999b). Sam therefore suggests that Sue may wish to explore leadership theory, linked to management of change and reflect on her leadership approach before she embarks on her plan.

Leadership of change

The pace of change within the healthcare environment is increasing and the challenges faced by the healthcare profession are huge and often difficult (Jooste, 2004; Sieloff, 2004). Sue notes from her research that in leading change it is suggested that the role of a leader is to act as a visionary; someone who assists 'employees to plan, organise, lead and control their activities' (Jooste, 2004:218) and that the qualities required of a leader in the current environment are less about power and authority and more concerned with how to 'motivate, persuade, appreciate, understand and negotiate' (Jooste, 2004:218). This approach resonates with Kotter's eight-step model of change, so Sue decides to investigate transformational leadership, a leadership style that encompasses this approach to managing change.

Transformational leadership, originally developed by MacGregor Burnes, occurs when leaders are able to appeal to 'followers' values that go beyond their personal interests (Grint, 2010). Transformational leaders are said to possess qualities that are needed 'to inspire and redirect staff to solve problems and attain ambitious objectives' (Knights and Willmott, 2007:281). Jooste (2004) suggests that it is an empowering leadership style, one which is highly suited to the nursing profession, the profession being characterised as caring and ethical in approach. The characteristics of this leadership style include being able to provide a compelling vision, to stimulate creativity and innovation, to link strategy to vision and to be able to communicate with, and persuade, others. The transformational leader is confident and optimistic (Mullins, 2010).

This change initiative, like many within the NHS, will be dependent upon the members of the ward team, and the multiprofessional team, being able to work together. It is suggested that in order to allow the team to work together and be innovative in its approaches a transformational leadership style is required (Outhwaite, 2003). This is because it will facilitate the empowerment of team members as they participate in, and lead, working groups aligned to their own areas of specialism and interest (Outhwaite, 2003).

However, in a change initiative, such as the change that Sue wishes to implement, it is important to maintain relationships with all those involved in, and affected by, the change process through two-way communication and the exchange of information and ideas (Flesner *et al.*, 2005:37) and in this respect transformational leaders recognise 'that building relationships among employees and departments is an essential component in transforming a work environment' (Flesner *et al.*, 2005:37).

A guide, *The Nursing Roadmap for Quality* (DH, 2010b) aims to provide a quality framework for healthcare professionals. This framework sets out seven key elements, including leadership for quality and is explored further in the next section.

Summary

In summary, when implementing change it is important to:

- Act as a visionary in communicating the required change.
- Motivate, persuade and inspire people to think and act beyond their personal interests.
- Stimulate creativity and innovation amongst employees/teams.
- Encourage participation and involvement in change, for example, through team working.
- Maintain relationships with all those involved in, and affected by, the change.

Using Government policy guidance to help implement evidence-based practice

---

Scenario

Sue and Sam are writing one of the final chapters of their dissertation; it asks them to consider some of the aspects of implementing evidence in practice. One of their lecturers has asked then to read some of the work of the former English Chief Nurse, Professor Christine Beasley, but, in particular, *The Nursing Roadmap for Quality* (DH, 2010b) and *High Impact Actions for Nursing and Midwifery: The Essential Collection* (http://www.institute.nhs.uk/building_capability/general/aims/). Both of these English health department documents are useful in helping nurses and others understand some of the aspects of implementing evidence-based practice. Sue and Sam have been able to download the documents form the department website.

Nurses are the guardians of much of the quality agenda which has emanated from the Department of Health in recent years. In 2008, Lord Darzi published *High Quality Care for All*. This was the final report of the NHS Next Stage Review (http://www.dh.gov.uk/en/Healthcare/Highquality careforall/index.htm). Simultaneously, the Department of Health published *Framing the Nursing and Midwifery Contribution* (DH, 2008), which summarised the contribution of nurses and midwives to Darzi's vision of a reformed health service.

The nursing contribution to quality enhancement

In March 2010, to help nurses engage in the drive for quality improvement as envisaged in these and other policy publications, the former English chief nursing officer, Professor Dame Christine Beasley, launched *The Nursing Roadmap for Quality* (DH, 2010b). This guide is aimed at helping nurses understand the various tools that are available for them to both measure and improve the quality of care they deliver. As nurses play a large part in almost all aspects of health service delivery, the chief nursing officer's 'roadmap' or quality framework set out seven key elements where she believed the profession can make a real difference:

1 Bringing clarity to quality
2 Measuring quality
3 Publishing quality performance
4 Recognising and rewarding quality
5 Leadership for quality
6 Safeguard quality
7 Staying ahead.

Nurses are required, as a reflection of their state registration and as governed by the NMC Code (NMC, 2008), to reaffirm the implicitness of their obligations to society in delivering high quality and compassionate care based on best evidence. (NB: other healthcare professions have similar codes.)

The NMC believes that in order to justify that trust to the public nurses must:

1 make the care of people your first concern, treating them as individuals and respecting their dignity;
2 work with others to protect and promote the health and wellbeing of those in your care, their families and carers, and the wider community;
3 provide a high standard of practice and care at all times;
4 be open and honest, act with integrity and uphold the reputation of your profession.

The former chief nurses 'roadmap' complements the NMC code and is precise in what nurses need to do to achieve the quality outcomes expected of them in tomorrow's NHS. Hence, it signposts the existing quality tools that nurses can use in their quest to help support quality improvements against the seven elements of the quality framework. Additionally, the roadmap gives readers access to a range of key resources, 41 in total, which they can use to enhance the nurses contribution to quality and in particular reduce waste and repetition through embracing the quality and productivity challenge of the reformation of the health service.

What are the implications of the roadmap for the nursing and other healthcare professions?

Registered practitioners such as nurses are at the heart of the NHS and have always been pivotal in the provision of high quality healthcare. Such professionals should be able to harness their professional power and their potential to improve the experiences of patients and influence the standards of care in all NHS settings. The nursing professions commitment to high quality care will help ensure continued public trust in their service provision. Given the key role and numerical status of nurses as a percentage of healthcare workforces, they are well placed to become champions of care in hospitals and the community's in which they work.

All healthcare professionals need to see quality through the perceptions of service users and ask the following allegorical questions on their behalf:

• Will I be safe?
• How effective will my treatment or care be?
• What will my experience of healthcare be like?

The 41 resources available through the roadmap framework for practitioners to use in answering these questions, allow them to tell their 'quality stories' in a meaningful and tangible way, thus facilitating transparency of care which can be shared among the healthcare professions. Some of these tools and resources can be used for the auditing and benchmarking of care practice and others can be used for specific measurement.

Bringing clarity to quality

Nurses and others need to be clear about the standards of care they expect their patients to receive. Quality standards pertinent to care and best evidence to underpin practice can be found at various sites such as The National Institute for Clinical excellence (http://www.nice.org.uk/) or The Royal College of Nursing (http://www.rcn.org.uk/).

Measuring quality

It is important that nurses and other healthcare professionals collect collate and interpret information about their care delivery to patients in order to drive up quality based on best evidence. This entails measurements and comparison with other teams or departments. The *Nursing Roadmap to Quality* gives details of a range of indicators nurses and others can use to measure their quality performance, such as *Essence of care: benchmarks for the care environment*, which is intended for all staff groups caring for patients across all organizations and settings (http://www.dh.gov.uk/en/Publicationsandstatistics/Publications/PublicationsPolicyAndGuidance/DH_080058). Additionally, tools to capture the voice of service users, such as the NHS National Patient Survey (http://www.nhssurveys.org/), are also highlighted. Soliciting the view of service users is now a mandatory requirement for care providers.

Publishing quality performance

In publishing accounts of quality activities nurses and other professional care groups can help disseminate good practice to the workforce as a whole. This can be undertaken in a variety of formats, not least being through healthcare journal editors, who are always interested in publishing papers which demonstrate good practice.

Leadership for quality

It is recognised that robust professional leadership is essential for the delivery of quality improvements in the NHS. The care a patient receives is only as good as the nurse or healthcare professional who delivers it. Professionals who lead teams of other professionals are crucially important and worthy of significant investment. Leadership courses for nurses and other healthcare professionals are available in most university faculties' of health.

Safeguarding quality

The Care Quality Commission (CQC) is the body trusted with regulating health and social care in England. The other countries of the United Kingdom have similar arrangements, for example, Audit Scotland (http://www.audit-scotland.gov.uk/careers/about.php).

In England, all NHS Trusts have to provide the CQC with data which show that they are compliant with their essential standards of care (Glasper, 2010b) (http://www.cqc.org.uk/newsandevents/newsstories.cfm?cit_id=34929& FAArea1=customWidgets.content_view_1&usecache=false).

Nurses and other healthcare professionals can play a major role in helping healthcare providers source the evidence they need to show compliance to the essential standards of care expected by healthcare regulators and, importantly, design initiatives to address issues of non-compliance when necessary. The former chief nurses' roadmap gives a full range of websites that point the way to tools to help practitioners safeguard quality in their workplace.

Activity

Download *The Nursing Roadmap for Quality* (DH, 2010b) and discuss its implications in your learning group (http://www.dh.gov.uk/en/Publicationsandstatistics/ Publications/PublicationsPolicyAndGuidance/DH_113450).

Can high impact nursing actions result in enhanced patient care?

In July 2010, the English government published its NHS White Paper and with it an indicator of the major changes to healthcare. In recognising the powerful changes to come in the delivery of health services, the former Chief Nursing Officer for England, Professor Christine Beasley, through the Institute for Innovation and Improvement published *High Impact Actions for Nursing and Midwifery: The Essential Collection*, which spotlighted eight excellent case studies from around the UK that were designed to highlight innovation in care delivery whilst simultaneously saving millions in healthcare expenditure (http://www.institute.nhs.uk/building_capability/general/ aims/).

The chief nurse's publication was timely, as contemporary healthcare delivery focuses on personalised care that reflects individuals' own health and care needs, supports carers and encourages strong joint arrangements and local partnerships The chief nurse's Essential Collection of case studies continues to highlights good examples of some of the innovative work which has been being undertaken by the nursing profession and others to improve the quality of care whilst also significantly reducing costs. The case studies endeavour to show professionals how to achieve such changes. The Essential Collection was designed to offer opportunities to help pave the way in delivering better care at lower cost.

How can the Essential Collection help healthcare practitioners to achieve quality enhancement?

Perhaps the key message of the chief nurse's collection of case studies was and continues to be the emphasis on measurement and a reinforcement of the old adage cited by National Patient Safety Agency 'that in God we trust. All others must bring data' (http://www.patientsafetyfirst.nhs.uk/ashx/Asset.ashx?path=/Press-releases/FINAL%20-%20Measurement%20Release%20-%2014th%20April%2009.pdf). The use by the nursing profession of patient data expressed in statistical terms goes back to the time of Nightingale who, in the nineteenth century when research reports were only beginning to include data expressed in table format, was pioneering the use of colour-coded bar and polar area diagrammatic pie charts to underpin significant findings, for example, deaths of soldiers from infection during the Crimean war. As a nurse, Nightingale took great pains to make the science of her findings comprehensible to readers. In particular, McDonald (2001) discusses how Nightingale used statistics to highlight the benefits to patient care of a trained nursing workforce compared to that of untrained pauper nurses.

Hence, a central tenet to the chief nurse's collection is measurement. All healthcare professionals, irrespective of their fields of practice, are involved in collecting data, ranging from clinical measurements of, for example, patient blood pressure, to weekly hand hygiene audits to ensure compliance to hospital protocols. It is important to stress that data are collected to help in informed decision making and good measurement is believed to enhance better decision making in all aspects of healthcare. Furthermore, all healthcare institutions providing services for the National Health Service are now required to publish data in the form of an annual quality account to underpin the quality of the services they provide to the public. Given the strategic importance of healthcare professionals to the whole operating framework of the NHS, it is they who play a large part in collecting and interpreting this mandatory data.

It is not sufficient to either know or understand the theory of what makes things better for patients but to actually go out and make them better. This was Professor Beasley's mission in publishing the Essential Collection, which highlights a number of criteria necessary for making a difference to patient care through *measurement*.

Developing a model for improvement

The PDSA model cited earlier (Plan, Do, Study, Act) or the 'rapid cycle change approach' has been used in manufacturing since the 1930s as a way of improving productivity and quality output. It is a simple but effective method for focusing on making improvements to patient delivery services.

Importantly, it allows nursing teams to be crystal clear in what they are proposing to implement and how to ensure that the proposals actually work in the practice setting. The PDSA cycle is facilitated through the posing of three specific questions:

1 What is it that the healthcare team is trying to accomplish? When setting goals to achieve the planned change, teams need to use objectives which are specific, achievable, realistic and time bound (SMART).

2 How will the team know that any change it makes is an improvement over the previous model? This stage in the PDSA cycle is all about measurement. The Essential Collection gives 'seven steps to measurement', which is a process practitioners have found useful when wishing to measure the effectiveness of any change to patient care or practice.

3 What changes can the team make to ensure that there is an improvement?

The Essential Collection gives real tangible examples of how professionals have made a difference to patient care. The chief nurse's publication gives details of how practitioners can use cause and effect or 'driver diagrams' to understand how the PDSA model of improvement can be articulated in the real world of practice. Nurses and others will be familiar with driver diagrams, as they resemble algorithms in which all the actions necessary to achieve the goal are visually laid out.

Driver diagrams can be used to conceptualise a clinical problem needing a solution and allow professionals to determine the individual components that need to be considered to develop the pathway to achieve the primary mission parameters or goals.

Activity

A good example of a driver diagram can be accessed at http://www.patient safetyalliance.scot.nhs.uk/docs/presentations/MedicinesManagementDriver Diagram.pdf.

Additionally, this Scottish Patient Safety Programme Medicines Management Driver Diagram and Change Package shows how professionals can provide safe and effective medicines management and reduce adverse drug events.

Is it all worthwhile?

Perhaps the final check point in the cycle of change is the need for teams to assess the return on their investment. Clearly there is an expectation that the planned outcomes are worthy of the cost of implementation, expressed in many forms and not just financial. Although not all improvement changes can be quantified in terms of cost savings, other criteria, such as improved quality of life, should be carefully documented as benefits resulting from service improvements. Healthcare professionals need to be able to show that any improvements they make which leads to enhanced quality care are also a better use of healthcare resources.

Advice on how to calculate returns on investments (ROI's) can be accessed via www.institute.nhs.uk/roi

The key themes in the Essential Collection of Case Studies

Clearly one of the roles of the chief nurse is to motivate and provide leadership to the whole of the nursing profession (and others) in its quest to drive up quality. In addition to project management there are some key themes which therefore must be addressed to ensure the success of PDSA projects. The first of these among others is communication and this concept features in all the Essential Collection of Case Studies. New and radical ways of communicating information and data are essential if the message is to be heard. A model of change in which communication features prominently is the social movement model. This model relies on coordinated activity which helps develop shared responsibilities in which groups of professionals can achieve bottom-up, locally led grass roots movements for improvement and change. (Bate *et al.*, 2004). The NHS Institute estimates that currently 15–20% of NHS staff is engaged in quality improvement work in order to try and meet the goals as set out in the various healthcare policies; however, it believes that the achievement of these goals may require 80–100% of staff engagement. Achieving this can be facilitated through a better understanding of, and buy-in to, social movement. *The Power of One, the Power of Many* (http://www.institute.nhs.uk/index.php?option=com_joomcart& Itemid=194&main_page=document_product_info&products_id=580) shows how social movement can be incorporated into contemporary healthcare improvement strategies.

It is vitally important where appropriate that healthcare professionals tangibly involve users in any improvement initiative and the case studies give good examples of how this can be achieved. It is important to stress, however, that perhaps none of the cited case studies in the Essential Collection would have succeeded without executive sponsorship. In a poignant example of how sponsorship and the power of one, the power of many can motivate the whole workforce, one chief executive in one of the featured healthcare institutions within the case studies states 'we have 6000 members of our infection control team – that's every member of our staff'.

Conclusion

Sue and Sam have been able to access these publications from the former chief nurses The Essential Collection is available by request by visiting http://www.institute.nhs.uk/HIA.

References

Alfaro-LeFevre, R. (2004) *Critical Thinking and Clinical Judgment A Practical Approach* (3rd edn). Saunders, Philadelphia, PA.

Allen, J., Jimmieson, N.L., Bordia, P. and Irmer, B.E. (2007) Uncertainty during organisational change: managing perceptions through communication. *Journal of Change Management*, **7** (2), 187–210.

Anderson, S. (2002) Managing Change: theory and evidence. *Journal of Clinical Evidence*, **4**, 339–341.

Anthony, P. (1994) *Managing Culture*. Open University Press, Buckingham, UK.

Arbon, P. (2004) Understanding experience in nursing. *Journal of Clinical Nursing*, **13**, 150–157.

Bate, P., Robert, G. and Bevan, H. (2004) The next phase of healthcare improvement: what can we learn from social movements? *Quality & Safety in Health Care*, **13**, 62–66.

Berragan, L. (1998) Nursing practice draws upon several different ways of knowing *Journal of Clinical Nursing*, **7**, 209–217.

Bower, F.L. (2000) *Nurses taking the lead Personal qualities of effective leadership*. W.B. Saunders Company, London.

Buckwalter, K.C., Grey, M., Bowers, B. *et al.* (2009) Intervention research in highly unstable environments. *Research in Nursing and Health*, **32**, 110–121.

Bullock, R.J. and Batten, D. (1985) It's Just a Phase We're Going Through: A Review and Synthesis of OD Phase Analysis. *Group Organisation Management*, **10** (4), 383–412.

Burnes, B. (2000) *Managing Change. A strategic approach to organizational dynamics* (3rd edn). Pearson Education Ltd, Harlow, UK.

Burns, N. and Grove, S. (2009) *The Practice of Nursing Research: Appraisal, Synthesis, and Generation of Evidence* (6th edn). Saunders, St. Louis.

Cullum, N. (2000) Users' guides to the nursing literature: an introduction. *Evidence-Based Nursing*, **3**, 71–72. DOI: 10.1136/ebn.3.3.71.

Cameron, E. and Green, M. (2009) *Making Sense of Change Management* (2nd edn). Kogan Page, London.

Carper, B.A. (1978) Fundamental Patterns of Knowing in Nursing. *Advances in Nursing Science*, **1** (1), 13–23.

Crosswaite, C. and Curtice, L. (1994) Disseminating research results – the challenge of bridging the gap between health research and health action. *Health Promotion International*, **9** (4), 289–296.

DH (Department of Health) (1993) *A Vision for the Future*. The Stationery Office, London.

DH (Department of Health) (1999a) *The NHS Plan*. The Stationery Office, London.

DH (Department of Health) (1999b) *Making a Difference: strengthening the nursing, midwifery and health visiting contribution to health and healthcare*. The Stationery Office, London.

DH (Department of Health) (2008) Framing the Nursing and Midwifery Contribution: driving up the quality of care. The Stationery Office, London (http://www.nipec. hscni.net/docs/driving_up_quality_care.pdf; accessed 20 June 2012).

DH (Department of Health) (2010a) *Equity and excellence: Liberating the NHS*. The Stationery Office, London.

DH (Department of Health) (2010b) *The Nursing Roadmap for Quality*. The Stationery Office, London (http://www.dh.gov.uk/en/Publicationsandstatistics/Publications/ PublicationsPolicyAndGuidance/DH_113450, accessed 25 May 2012).

Dunn, E.V., Norton, P.G., Stewart, M., Tudiver, F. and Bass, M.J. (1994) *Disseminating Research/Changing Practice*, Volume 6. Sage Publications, London.

Fineout-Overholt, E. and Melnyk, B. (2005) Building a culture of best practice. *Nurse Leader*, **3** (6), 26–30.

Flesner, M.K., Scott-Cawiezell, J. and Rantz, M. (2005) Preparation of nurse leaders in the 21st century workplace. *Nurse Leader*, **3** (4), 37–40.

Glasper, A. (2010a) Can high-impact nursing actions result in enhanced patient care? *British Journal of Nursing*, **19** (16), 1016–1057.

Glasper, A. (2010b) The Care Quality Commission Criteria for assessing NHS Trusts. *British Journal of Nursing*, **19** (5), 280–281.

Gordon, M. (1980) Predictive strategies in diagnostic tasks. *Nursing Research*, **29**, 39–45.

Greenhalgh, T. (2006) *How to read a paper. The basics of evidence-based medicine* (3rd edn). Blackwell Publishing, Oxford.

Grint, K. (2010) *Leadership. A very short introduction*. Oxford University Press, Oxford.

Harding, T.A. and Sque, M. (2010) Do Leadership Skills Impact Clinical Decisions Made by Ward Managers? *Nurse Leader*, **8** (1), 42–45.

Hedberg, B. and Satterlund Larsson. U. (2003) Observations, confirmations and strategies – useful tools in decision-making process for nurses in practice? *Journal of Clinical Nursing*, **12**, 215–222.

Higgins, J.M. (1991) *The management challenge: An introduction to management*. McMillan, London.

Holt, J., Barrett, C. and Monks, R. (2000) The globilization of nursing knowledge. *Nurse Education Today*, **20**, 426–431.

Hussey, P.S., Anderson, G.F., Osborn, R. *et al.* (2004) How Does the Quality of Care Compare in Five Countries? *Health Affairs*, **23** (3), 89–99. DOI: 10.1377/ hlthaff.23.3.89.

Johns, C. (2003) Clinical supervision as a model for leadership. *Journal of Advanced Management*, **11**, 25–34.

Jooste, K. (2004) Leadership a new perspective. *Journal of Nursing Management*, **12**, 217–223.

Kitson, A., Harvey, G. and McKormack, B. (1998) Approaches to implementing research in practice. *Quality in Health Care*, **7**, 149–159.

Knights, D. and Willmott, H. (2007) *Introducing Organisational Behaviour and Management*. Thomson Learning, London.

Kotter, J.P. (1995) Leading Change: Why transformation efforts fail. *Harvard Business Review*, **73** (2), 59–67.

Lacey, E.A. (1994) Research utilisation in nursing practice – a pilot study. *Journal of Advanced Nursing*, **19**, 987–995.

Leeman, J., Baernholdt, M. and Sandelowski, M. (2007) Developing a theory-based taxonomy of methods for implementing change in practice. *Journal of Advanced Nursing*, **58** (2), 191–200.

Lines, R. (2004) Influence of participation in strategic change: resistance, organisational commitment and change goal achievement. *Journal of Change Management*, **4** (3), 193–215.

McCormack, B., Kitson, A., Harvey, G., Rycroft-Malone, J., Titchen, A. and Seers, K. (2002) Getting Evidence into Practice: the meaning of 'context'. *Journal of Advanced Nursing*, **38** (1), 94–104.

McDonald, L. (2001) Florence Nightingale and the early origins of evidence based nursing. *Evidence Based Nursing*, **4**, 68–69.

McGlynn, E.A., Asch, S.M., Adams, J. *et al.* (2003) The Quality of Health Care Delivered to Adults in the United States. *New England Journal of Medicine*. **348**, 2635–2645.

Mullins, L.J. (2010) *Management and Organisational Behaviour* (9th edn). Pearson Education Ltd, Harlow, UK.

Nelson, D.L., and Quick, J.C. (2011) *Principles of Organisational Behaviour. Realities and Challenges*, 8th edn. Cengage Learning (South-Western College Publishing), UK.

Nemeth, L.S. (2003) Implementing Change for Effective Outcomes. *Outcomes Management*, **7** (3), 134–139.

NHS Centre for Reviews and Dissemination (1999) Getting Evidence into Practice. *Effective Health Care*, **5** (1), 1–16.

NMC (2008) The Code: Standards of conduct, performance and ethics for nurses and midwives. Nursing and Midwifery Council, London.

Oermann, M.H., Nordstrom, C.K., Wilmes, N.A., *et al.* (2008) Dissemination of research in clinical nursing journals. *Journal of Clinical Nursing*, **17** (2), 149–156.

Offredy, M. (1998) The application of decision making concepts by nurse practitioners in general practice. *Journal of Advanced Nursing*, **28** (5), 998–1000.

Outhwaite, S. (2003) The importance of leadership in the development of an integrated team. *Journal of Nursing Management*, **11**, 371–376.

Parahoo, K. (2006) *Nursing Research: Principles, Process and Issues* (2nd edn). Palgrave Macmillan, Houndmills.

Pinch, W.J. (2001) Improving patient care through the use of research. *Orthopaedic Nursing*, **20** (4), 75.

Redelmeier, D.A., Ferris, L.E., Tu, J.V., Hux, J.E. and Schull, M.J. (2001) Problems for clinical judgement: introducing cognitive psychology as one more basic science. *Canadian Medical Association Journal*, **164** (3), 358–360.

Robbins, S.P. (2001) *Organizational Behavior* (9th edn). Prentice Hall International, Inc., NJ.

Rollinson, D. (2008) *Organisational Behaviour and Analysis. An integrated approach* (4th edn). Pearson Education Ltd, Harlow, UK.

Russ, T.L. (2008) Communicating Change: A review and critical analysis of programmatic and participatory implementation approaches. *Journal of Change Management*, **8** (3/4), 199–211.

Rycroft-Malone, J., Kitson, A., Harvey, G. *et al.* (2002). Ingredients for Change: revisiting a conceptual framework. *Quality Safe Health Care*, **11**, 174–180.

Rycroft-Malone, J., Seers, K., Titchen, A., Harvey, G., Kitson, A. and McCormack, B. (2004) What counts as evidence-based practice? *Journal of Advanced Nursing*, **47** (1), 81–90.

Sackett, D.L., Rosenberg, W.M.C., Muir Gray, J.A., Haynes, R.B. and Richardson, W.S. (1996) Evidence based medicine. What it is and what it isn't. *British Medical Journal*, **312**, 71–72.

Sheldon, L.K. and Ellington, L. (2008) Application of a model of social information processing to nursing theory: how nurses respond to patients. *Journal of Advanced Nursing*, **64** (4), 388–398. (Article first published online: September 2008. DOI: 10.1111/j.1365-2648.2008.04795.x.)

Sieloff, C.L. (2004) Leadership behaviours that foster nursing group power. *Journal of Nursing Management*, **12**, 246–251.

Stetler, C.B. (2003) Role of the Organisation in Translating Research into Evidence-Based Practice. *Outcomes Management*, **7** (3), 97–103.

Teal, T. (1998) cited in *Harvard Business Review on Leadership*. Harvard Business Review Press, Boston.

Thomas, P. (1985) *The Aims and Outcomes of Social Policy Research*. Crook Helm, London.

Thompson, C. and Dowding, D. (2002) *Clinical Decision Making and Judgement in Nursing*. Churchill Livingston, London.

Tod, A., Palfreyman, S. and Burke, L. (2004) Evidence-based practice is a time of opportunity for nursing. *British Journal of Nursing*, **13** (4), 211–216.

Torrington, D., Hall, L. and Taylor, S. (2002) *Human Resource Management* (5th edn). Financial Times Prentice Hall, Harlow, UK.

Veeramah, V. (2004) Utilisation of research findings by graduate nurses and midwives. *Journal of Advanced Nursing*, **47**, 183–191.

Wilson, D. (1992) *A Strategy of Change*. Routledge, London.

Young, A.P. and Cooke, M. (2002) *Managing and Implementing Decisions in Health Care*. Bailliere Tindall, London.

For further resources for this chapter visit the companion website at
www.wiley.com/go/glasper/nursingdissertation

Section 7   **Taking your dissertation further: disseminating evidence, knowledge transfer; writing as a professional skill**

Sam has been asked to present a poster based on his dissertation for a forthcoming hospital conference. Sue wants to write a paper for publication in a well-known national nursing journal.

Chapter 21   Publishing your dissertation: In a journal or at a conference

John Fowler[1] and Colin Rees[2]
[1]*Sheffield Hallam University, UK*
[2]*Cardiff University,* UK

Scenario

Sue and Sam were really pleased when they had completed their dissertations. They had worked hard and this represented a real achievement. They both did well and their dissertation supervisor said to each of them they should think about presenting their dissertation at a local conference and maybe publish it in a journal.

Your dissertation is complete: what next?

If you, like Sue and Sam, have now completed your dissertation and you are quite pleased with your grade, what is your next step? You have three options:

1 Do nothing; enjoy the well-earned rest. Put your dissertation and degree on the bookshelf and let the dust begin to gather!

2 You can try and adapt your dissertation for publication in a suitable journal. This is quite achievable, although it is not as easy as it might initially appear. You will probably need the equivalent of at least a week's work to convert a standard dissertation to an article suitable for publication.

3 You can submit an abstract of your dissertation, or an aspect of it, for consideration at a suitable conference. This is also quite achievable. It will take approximately one day's work to complete the abstract and, if accepted for presentation at the conference, about another three day's work to prepare the conference presentation paper.

How to Write Your Nursing Dissertation, First Edition. Alan Glasper and Colin Rees.
© 2013 John Wiley & Sons, Ltd. Published 2013 by John Wiley & Sons, Ltd.

The first option is very tempting, particularly after working hard for a number of years on your degree. However, we would encourage you to consider either or both of options two and three. The very nature of a degree and especially a master's degree is the recognition that you have moved beyond being a student. You now have something to share; something to teach others in your discipline. By virtue of finishing your degree you have demonstrated not only commitment to your subject but also that you can manage time and complete work to a deadline. Most healthcare professionals complete Master's degrees whilst at the same time working clinically and maintaining family commitments. So why stop just because your degree is finished?

Motivation

So what is the first and most important step in getting your dissertation ready for a conference presentation or publication in a journal? It is not the quality of the critical analysis or the general quality of the writing within your dissertation. Neither is it the grade you received from the university. Whilst these are important factors in academic writing and are relevant in published work and conference presentations, they are not the most important factor in moving your work on from completed dissertation to potential conference presentation or publication. The most important factor in getting your work more widely recognised is your drive or motivation to take it forward. If you do not really want to get your work more widely recognised then the first knock-back will stop you, and your dissertation will remain on the bookcase gathering dust.

So what motivates and drives people to publish their work or present it at a conference, to put in that additional effort?

For some of you it may be part of your role. If you fail to achieve a certain number of publications or conference publications then your job is in jeopardy! As you can imagine, this is a strong motivator. It is one that drives a number of research academics in university departments. University departments are rated on the quality and quantity of research conferences and publications and this rating attracts considerable funding, hence the drive.

For others, the motivation for taking your dissertations forward is that you want your CV to reflect this level of work and achievement. If you intend applying for a clinical nurse specialist role, a nurse consultant post or a university lecturer post you will be at an advantage if you have conference presentations and publications on your CV. If I was interviewing anyone who had completed a dissertation-based degree, I would almost certainly be asking what they subsequently did with their dissertation. The candidate that answers positively is at a great advantage.

Another factor that may motivate you is a simple ambition to present at a national conference or publish in a professional journal, maybe for your family or, often, just to prove to yourself that you can do it.

Some of you, often those who work in specialist areas, will have an aspect of practice that you have developed as part of your dissertation and you wish to share that with others. This is something that you feel very strongly about. What better way than at a conference of people all interested in that particular area of practice.

Finally, there are those people who just want to see their name in print, either in a journal or in a conference handbook.

Conference abstract and presentation

Writing a conference abstract

This is the first and most important step in presenting your work at a conference. There are many nursing conferences each year covering all varieties of clinical speciality, a number of educational conferences, some specifically researched-based ones and some quite unusual fringe conferences. Whatever your subject, you can be sure there is a conference that would welcome a well constructed abstract regarding your potential paper. This section will consider the following aspects of writing a conference abstract:

- Choosing the right conference
- Local, national or international conference
- Presenting all or some of your dissertation
- Following the conference committees abstract guidelines and general structure of the abstract
- Formulating the title and creating interest
- Submission procedure.

Choosing the right conference

There are a large number of nursing and healthcare conferences held each year. These vary according to clinical speciality, education based, research conferences, reflective practice and an array of alternative aspects of healthcare. Some conferences are very local, organised by a hospital Trust and targeting the local population. Others are nationally focussed and others are international. So which one is right for you? Unlike potential publications to a journal, with conference abstracts you can submit the same or a very similar abstract to different conferences. However, this is not to be recommended. It is far better to research the various conferences, assess them according to various criteria and then make a focused abstract application. So what sort of criteria should you be exploring when considering which conference to submit your abstract to? Consider:

1 What date is the conference? Would you be free to attend the conference? This sounds obvious and very 'non-academic' but it is always the first thing to consider. The conference advert for abstracts usually comes out about 10 months prior to the actual conference, but even with that notice you may have something more important in your diary. So make sure you are free to attend the conference and then pencil that date in your diary.

2 Is the conference advert asking for subjects that relate to your dissertation topic? If not, could some aspect of your dissertation be adapted to one of the themes of the conference.

3 Is your dissertation at the right sort of level for that particular conference? If you have undertaken a relatively small study in one ward using six interviews, then it is unlikely that the 'International Conference of Advanced Nursing Research' would consider your work. Choose a conference that appears to want your style and level of dissertation. If you are unsure then discuss it with a more experienced colleague who may have been to similar conferences.

4 Where is the conference and would you be able to get funding to attend. You are more likely to get support and funding to attend a conference that is being held 30 miles away, is for one day only and costs £50 to attend rather than for an international conference, the other side of the world, lasting for four days and costing over a thousand pounds. Most conferences will expect presenters to pay the conference fee and cover their own travelling and accommodation costs.

Local, national or international conference

As you can see from the above, the implications of applying to present at an international conference are significant in terms of cost and travel. If you have undertaken a funded research project then the cost of results dissemination in terms of conference presentations may have been incorporated into the costing of the research. Other people search the various adverts that appear in the nursing and healthcare journals that offer support for international travel. Occasionally, your local Trust or employer will have special trust funds that have been set aside from legacies to support such travel. It is certainly worth exploring the various options for funding.

Presenting all or some of your dissertation

A dissertation normally has sections on: underpinning literature, methodology, sampling technique, data analysis, findings, conclusions and implications for practice. A conference presentation does not need to cover all of these. Indeed it would be very difficult to do justice to all of these in the standard 20-minute slot that most conferences allocate to such presentations. Your abstract, however, should give a brief overview of these aspects and then identify your particular focus of the presentation. If you have a lot of data that can be analysed from different perspectives then you may choose to focus on one particular area for a specific conference, for example, age, gender, ethnicity, grade of staff, hospital verses community and so on.

Following abstract guidelines

Each conference will publish guidelines regarding the structure, content and submission details for the conference abstract. It is very important that you follow the specific guidelines exactly. They generally give you a word limit of approximately 500 words and ask for details which require you to do the following:

1 Identify where your presentation fits into the structure and subthemes of the conference as presented in their guidelines.
2 Present the theoretical and clinical background which gives context to your work.
3 Identify the methodology or the style of your study, for example 'a survey of 300 staff nurses from one Trust using purposive sampling to represent all wards'.
4 Identify the way in which the data were or are to be analysed.
5 What are the objectives of the study?
6 What if any are the interim findings?
7 Then return to the bigger picture as to how your findings might inform the theoretical and clinical areas identified in the first section above.

Formulating the title and creating interest

Conference abstracts, by their very nature, often appear factual but dull. The abstract that you submit, if accepted, will be the one that appears in the conference programme and the one that the conference delegates will use to make their choice of which presentations to attend. This needs to be borne in mind when writing your initial abstract. You have a very limited number of words, so use them to achieve two main objectives: firstly, to convey the quality of the presentation and, secondly, to instil a little intrigue into the readers mind. You can use the title quite effectively to do this. Review the following:

- The ups and downs in the life of Betty. A longitudinal case study of a patient diagnosed with a bipolar condition.
- Stress levels of clinical nurses: burn out or fade out!
- Nursing leadership: arc we herding sheep?
- Advanced nursing skills: the developing role of the HCA

Notice how you can use the title to convey precise meaning and also present it in a way that makes people want to read the abstract and attend the presentation.

Submission procedure

The submission of your conference abstract is usually electronic. The guidelines are very helpful but must be followed exactly, particularly the submission dates. Normally you receive an automated response saying you abstract has been received.

Members of the organising committee will review all of the abstracts submitted. Normally each abstract is given to two members of the committee who both make an independent assessment of its potential to be included in the conference. They will use some or all of the following criteria:

- Does the abstract conform to the published guidelines for the conference?
- Is it written and presented at a level consistent with the conference standing and reputation?
- Does the information appear valid and reliable?
- Does the abstract offer a new perspective on an established theory or practice?
- Does the abstract present new knowledge?
- Have there been a number of other similar abstracts covering the same topic?

Scenario

Sam submitted an abstract for a local conference and eight weeks later he received confirmation of its acceptance. He was both pleased and at the same time anxious as he now had to write his presentation.

Writing your conference presentation

Congratulations! Your conference abstract has been accepted; now you must write your conference presentation. The good news is that you normally have about four or five months between being notified that your abstract has been accepted and having to actually prepare your presentation. There are two ways that people prepare their presentations:

1 Some people write out verbatim exactly what it is they want to say. They time it to see how long it is going to take during many practice sessions and adjust content accordingly. They produce several pages of notes, often with accompanying PowerPoint® slides. The presentation has them

reading word for word their prepared 'lecture'. The advantage of this is that they cover exactly what they intend to cover; if they are nervous they just have to read their notes and there is no risk of them 'drying up'. The disadvantage to this, as we all know, is that this sort of presentation, even by the most learned people, is quite boring for the listener.

2   A second option is to prepare a number of trigger points; these can be PowerPoint slides or any other form of 'prop' and then talk through each of the trigger points, without using notes. To do this successfully you need to know your subject well and be confident enough to know you will not collapse at the front of the audience in a nervous and shaking wreck. The other disadvantage of this style is that it is difficult to keep to time, but the advantage is that your presentation is usually far more interesting, conveying not only information but passion and interest as well.

Pick the option that will work for you. If it helps, rather than seeing them as two distinct options, view them as a continuum and make your presentation somewhere in the middle. Whatever style you choose make sure you prepare thoroughly.

Writing a paper for publication

> **Scenario**
>
> Sue decides that she wants to try and publish her dissertation in a journal. She is tempted to just send it off to the journal that she subscribes to; but is that the best way forward?

The need to plan

Healthcare professionals, particularly clinically-based nurses, tend to be very action orientated people; they see something that needs doing and they get on and do it. These are admirable qualities but ones that need just a little holding back if you are to achieve successful publication of your dissertation. It is not just a matter of sending off your dissertation to a journal; that will almost certainly result in a rejection letter. Think of it like planning patients' care: a little time spent assessing needs and planning the way forward will produce better quality and more efficient practice and patient care. It is the same with publication.

Firstly you need to spend some time assessing the various journals and deciding which one is suitable for your work. Then you need to find, read and implement the authors' guidelines; this will help you produce a better quality article in a more efficient way. It will produce an article which is much more likely to be accepted for publication than if you had just jumped in and started writing without doing that preparation. The first thing to do is to make yourself familiar with a few copies of the journals that are relevant to your dissertation. Just flick through a few different journals and you will note the general style and variations in what they publish. Each journal is different.

Reviewing the guidelines: What will they tell you?

• General advice

This includes the type of article that the journal publishes and the particular readership that it targets. It will give you advice about headings, use of boxes, the referencing technique required and general layout of the article.

Have a look at the *British Journal of Nursing*'s 'Instructions to Authors'; these are particularly useful (http://www.britishjournalofnursing.com/contribute.shtml).

• Article structure

This includes the word length, the type of headings required, the style of language and the identification of key words. These vary considerably with different journals.

• Specialist journal advice

Journals which target a particular topic will often have quite specific advice. The *Journal of Clinical Nursing* has, for example, a large section on ethical guidelines (http://www.wiley.com/bw/submit.asp?ref=0962-1067&site=1).

• Different types of papers

Some journals are very specific regarding how particular papers are presented. The *Journal of Advanced Nursing*, for example, has different guidelines on eleven types of papers it publishes including 'systematic reviews', clinical trials, concept analysis and discussion papers (http://www.journalofadvanced nursing.com/default.asp?file=authorinfo).

Do not let this important planning stage of writing dampen your enthusiasm for publication. A little time spent choosing the appropriate journal and following their advice is time well spent. As a general rule the journal that you find most useful and interesting to read is the journal you should aim to publish your first article in.

Creating interest

Your dissertation has been written according to certain university standards and criteria. Your academic supervisor will have read and marked your dissertation because that is their job! Not necessarily because they found it intrinsically interesting. You now need to convert your dissertation into something other people will want to read. Think about your own reading habits. Which articles have you looked at in a journal recently and which of those articles, if any, did you go on to actually read? Your responses to these questions will differ to those of your colleagues but underpinning all the responses will be 'those that appeared interesting to me'. Consider what drew you to look at certain articles? It may be some or all of the following:

- The Title – Is the title intriguing? Is the topic one in which I am professionally or clinically interested in? Is this a subject that is currently in the news? Does the title suggest that I will be able to understand the content of the full article? If not I will probably ignore it.
- The Presentation – Is the article one big block of writing? Or is it broken up with headings, boxes, diagrams and possibly pictures?
- What do the headings say? Do they provoke interest?

Whether you do this consciously or not, you will be making similar judgements about each of the articles you look at and you will carry out that evaluation in about ten seconds. If during this initial scan something rings positive, then you will stop scanning and pay more attention. You will begin to selectively read bits of the article. It is unlikely that at this stage you will start at the first sentence and read every single sentence in order until you reach the end. For me it goes something like this:

I will start with the subtitle: the phrase that follows the main title and gives you a bit more information about the article.

Then I will have a go at the abstract: the collection of sentences right at the beginning that is meant to sum up the article, usually about 250 words. But I even find myself skip reading the abstract if the first sentence does not capture me.

At this stage, I will look in more detail at the boxes and pictures and I will scan the sections again to see if there is a particular part of the article that appeals more to me than others. Personally, I always read those short patient case studies that are often in boxes.

If at this stage I am convinced that this article has something more for me then I will read the conclusion, I will look at who has written it and make judgements as to what perspective they are coming from.

Finally, and to be honest, only rarely, will I return to the beginning and read the article through from beginning to end!

Now put yourself in the position of an author, it's the same, but in reverse. Firstly, you want to capture the reader's attention, then you want them to start scanning the article and, finally, you want to draw them into the main body of what you are saying. One way of doing this once you have written your article, is to put it to one side for a few days and then look at it again, but this time from a readers perspective; if it does not look interesting then refine it.

Targeting the right journal

Although I have been a nurse for over 30 years, I still discover nearly every week a journal that is related to health or nursing in some way that I have never heard of before. There is an enormous amount of journals out there to which you could potentially submit an article. How do you choose which one? Custom and general standards dictate that you do not submit your article to more than one journal at a time, so which one do you adapt your dissertation for? As the time between submission of an article and the editors response as to rejection or acceptance, is on average 8–12 weeks, you cannot afford to keep submitting your work to random journals in the hope that one of them will eventually accept it. In the same way that there are the five 'right' ways to give medication to patients, there are the four 'right' ways to get your dissertation published in the right journal:

- Right content – is the subject matter appropriate for the journal?
- Right level – what level have you written your dissertation at? Can you adapt it to the journal level?
- Right time – a topical subject is more likely to get accepted than one they have just run a series on.
- Right style – you need to adapt your writing style to that of the journal.

As a general rule, nursing and healthcare related journals target one of the following areas in their publication:

- A variety of clinical issues for all types of nurses; for example, the *British Journal of Nursing*.
- A specialist medical focus; for example, the *British Journal of Neuroscience Nursing*.
- A professional organisation's journal covering clinical, research and management, reaching the majority of its profession; for example, the *British Journal of Occupational Therapy*.
- An educational focus; for example, the *Nurse Education Today*.
- A management focus; for example, the *Journal of Health Care Management*.
- Weekly topical news and generic issues; for example, the *Nursing Times* or the *Nursing Standard*.

Secondly, journals can be categorised according to their 'research impact' factor. This is the importance that university research funding bodies associate with publications in certain journals. Thus, the *Journal of Advanced Nursing* is recognised as having a higher research impact factor than the *Nursing Times* or the *Journal of Nursing*.

Finally, journals can be viewed as to their 'readership impact', that is the number of nurses that actually read that journal. So, an article in the *Nursing Times* or *British Journal of Nursing* will be read by a far greater audience of clinically-based nurses than an article in one of the high impact research journals.

Thus, you are left with choices of where the article from your dissertation best fits in terms of the speciality of its subject matter, its level of originality and research base, who you want to read it and, finally, why you want it published. You may end up writing two articles from your dissertation for two different journals, one detailing the research base of your work and the second the more general application of your subject to the working staff nurse. If you are still unsure regarding which journal is appropriate for your work, then view the author guidelines for the potential journals and make sure you read some of the article published in these journals so that you are aware of the style and standard required.

One of the main skills of writing for a professional publication is to be organised: assess what, why and how you are going to write, and then submit it to the appropriate journal. As a note of caution, beware of online publications that charge you to publish your work. They may offer easy publication but the financial cost to you is often hidden in the small print.

Adapting a dissertation for publication

If Sue or you simply submit your complete dissertation or even a quickly edited version of it to a journal, then you will almost certainly receive a rejection letter. To understand this you need to think about the difference between a dissertation and an article in a journal.

What are the characteristics of a dissertation written for a university course?

The purpose of a dissertation is for the student to provide evidence that they demonstrate a degree of understanding of a specific subject. The dissertation will normally be grounded in the established literature. The student will be expected to show an understanding, discussion and critical analysis of this literature. Approximately 25% of the dissertation will be reviewing the published literature. The dissertation will then have sections or chapters on the methodology on which the dissertation was based, about 10% of the dissertation may be given over to this. Then there is a record of the actual research process: the ethical procedure, how sampling was established, data collection design and other practical implications relating to the dissertation. This may be another 10%. The results follow, which might take about 20% of the total, followed by discussion, another 20%. Finally, a conclusion which tries to embed the results and discussion back into the established literature, about 10%, with a final section on implications for future work and practice, about 5%. The dissertation is usually a minimum of 10 000 words for a Bachelor's degree, approximately 20 000 for a Master's degree and maybe 50 000 for a PhD.

What are the characteristics of an article written for professional publication?
- Most articles are between 2000 and 4000 words length.
- The purpose of an article is to communicate new ideas to someone who may or may not be interested in reading what you have to say.
- It is well presented and paragraphs are usually quite short.
- Headings are used to guide the reader into the subject.
- Approximately 10% of the article will be used to introduce the subject to the non-specialist reader.
- Approximately 20% of the article will reference the work to the underpinning literature.
- Approximately 70% of the article will be presenting new information or discussion and application of established knowledge.
- An article should be both informative and interesting to read.

The literature review

One of the big differences between writing a dissertation and converting it for publication is how you use the literature. The percentage of the written work given over to its review may be similar, around 20%, but in your article this translates to about 400 words. It is there to show the reader where this article 'fits' in terms of the established body of knowledge on the subject rather than demonstrate the breadth, debate and depth of analysis normally associated with a dissertation. In your article the literature review will normally be short, concise yet thorough. In an international journal it should reflect the international literature as well as the national literature. It should reflect an historical perspective and then locate the current thinking.

The body

Having established the theoretical underpinning of your work you then need to identify the body of your article. This should be introduced in a short, concise yet informative way that creates interest in the reader's mind. They should be left knowing the exact details of what you are writing about. Use numbers and precise language; for example, '*a change of practice on a 10 bedded unit after three weeks of planning*' or '*the development of a multidisciplinary care pathway for approximately 2000 patients a year with XYZ condition covering both community and hospital treatment*'.

Having introduced the main theme of the article you then need to say what it is that you have done, or discus a different perspective on something that has already been written about. A good article will also have two or three subthemes that weave through the body of your article. For example, if you were writing about the development of a care plan you may include as subthemes some of the following: finance, ethics, change management, infection control, patient satisfaction and so on. Having two or three subthemes to your article will help give it structure, depth, continuity and application. These can be drawn together in your conclusion, giving it structure, focus and challenge.

The conclusion and way forward
How does the body of your article relate to the underpinning literature? What themes have emerged and been developed? How does this impact on practice? What are the challenges in taking this work forward? What are your views?

You can begin to see how an article differs from that of your dissertation; whilst they both have a foundation of evidence as their base, their structure and presentation differ.

What will you do with your dissertation?

At the beginning of this chapter we presented you with three choices for you and your dissertation: put it on the shelf and let it and 'possibly you' gather dust; or look for a conference presentation within it; or adapt it or part of it for publication. Over the years I have probably worked with over 50 nurses and allied healthcare staff, helping them to publish an idea or a topic from their dissertation. None of those people have found it easy, none of those people have been given time off to write that article. The reason those people have succeeded is not because they are cleverer than others, or that their dissertation was at distinction level, it was because they were determined and hard working. Publication is about focus, effort and hard work. That is why a CV that includes conference presentations and publications as well as your clinical experience and expertise is so important when it comes to senior roles and your promotion; it demonstrates not only knowledge but application, commitment and hard work. Do not let the dust settle!

For further resources for this chapter visit the companion website at
www.wiley.com/go/glasper/nursingdissertation

Chapter 22 **Reflecting on your dissertation journey**

Wendy Wigley
University of Southampton, UK

'*Facts bring us to knowledge but stories bring us to wisdom*'
Rachel Naomi Remen (1997)

Scenario

Sue is writing the final elements of her dissertation. Her supervisor has reminded her that *she must include a section in her thesis on her reflection of her whole dissertation journey*. He has suggested she use a reflection model and she has a vague recollection of doing something similar during her initial training. Over coffee Sam, who has also included a reflective section in his own master's thesis, helps Sue understand the process.

Reflection

Christopher Johns has written widely about reflection in nursing and he describes reflection as a 'pool'. The pool has a shallow end, where the bottom is visible, and a deep end, where the blue is deep and the bottom unknown (Johns, 2004).

Reflection in nursing enables understanding of 'self' in context and application of theory to practice, as such reflection is a good way for Sue to explore *her individual and unique* experience of writing her dissertation because reflection is a method by which we can make sense of a situation, experience – good or bad – and begin to understand how we have learned because of (or in spite of) the situation or experience.

Sam explains that reflection is a process of self-development often used in vocational professions such as teaching and healthcare. Experts

---

How to Write Your Nursing Dissertation, First Edition. Alan Glasper and Colin Rees.
© 2013 John Wiley & Sons, Ltd. Published 2013 by John Wiley & Sons, Ltd.

> **Scenario**
>
> Sam explains how he feels about reflection: *'Like looking into a the deep end of the pool, reflection is about exploring elements of ourselves that we do not yet know. This way we can learn to know "self" better and in doing so learn to value all that we are and all that we would aspire to become, not only as a nurse but as a person'.*
> *'OK Sam'*, says Sue, *'that's all very good (if a bit "fluffy") … but what exactly is reflection?'*

on the process of reflection often talk about the 'self', 'self as nurse', 'self as teacher', 'self as student' and so on. Sue's supervisor wants Sue to be able to demonstrate what Sue has learnt about her 'self' during the dissertation journey, what were the good points and what went not so well. In short, a reflection tells the reader your story. Sam explains that his favorite description of reflection comes from Johns (2003) who describes it as *'thinking about thinking'.*

'OK', thinks Sue, *'but where does this sort of reflection originate from?'*

The forefather of reflection was John Dewey (1859–1952) a twentieth century American philosopher and psychologist who was a campaigner for changing the way in which children were taught. Dewey stated:

'We do not learn by doing … we learn by doing and realising what came of what we did …'

(Dewey, 1929, cited by Driscoll and Teh, 2001)

As such, Dewey saw education as a process of experience that required the application of thought.

Schon (1983) identified that nursing as a profession can potentially involve decision making activities that could be construed as messy; in other words, nurses often find it hard to explain their actions, what they do and why they do it. He described this as *knowing-in-action.*

However, when having to undertake a new or complex task, the practitioner has to think about what they are doing while they are doing it; Schon (1983) described this process as *reflection-in-action.* Sam explains that an example of *reflection-in-action* might be when Sue is explaining to a student colleague what she is doing when changing a patient's dressing. Perhaps without her colleague observing Sue would just change the dressing while chatting to the patient (*knowing-in-action*). When the colleague is present Sue has to recall, think about and explain her actions (while still chatting to the patient).

Reflection-on-action is a process that happens after the event. Using the example above Sam explains that *reflection-on-action* might involve Sue and her colleague sitting down together and formally recalling the process of the dressing change, it might involve the student colleague writing their own thoughts on the process, or Sue formally writing down what it felt like for her to explain the process to her colleague.

'*So do I just write down about how I felt about writing the dissertation?*' Sue asks Sam. '*Well you could*', Sam says, '*but so that this chapter is not just a ramble about how you felt … it would be easier for you to if you used a "framework"*'.

Frameworks for reflection

Sam explains to Sue that in nursing we are familiar with frameworks to guide our practice; for example, in the nursing process we *assess, plan, implement* and *evaluate* the care we provide to an individual or a group of clients. This framework (Figure 22.1) is often depicted as a cyclical process.

Frameworks are often called models, but basically they are methods which are designed to help us structure our thoughts and actions. Sam explains that we use frameworks in nursing to ensure that the care we give is based upon sound clinical judgement. Likewise, when we reflect we are making a judgement of ourselves in relation to an experience, in Sue's case writing her dissertation.

'*How do I choose a framework or model of reflection?*'

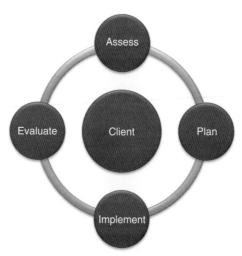

Figure 22.1   The nursing process.

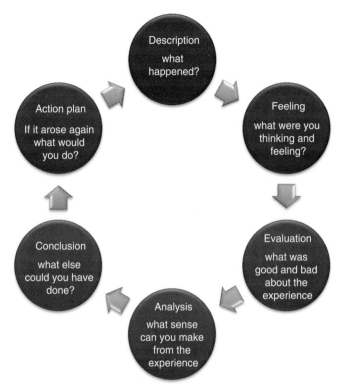

Figure 22.2   The Gibbs reflective cycle.

Sam explains that there are many models of reflection but often it is best to choose a model that seems to 'fit' with who you are as a person and how you like to think. Sam explains that the model Sue chooses should make her *really* think about what she has learnt from writing her dissertation. Some models are quite simple, others are more complex. Sam's opinion is that the more complex the model the 'deeper' you can explore your thoughts and, in doing so, the learning you have gained from the experience can also be critical and more analytical.

'*All well and good*', says Sue, '*can we start with a simple model*?'

Gibbs reflective cycle (1988)

The Gibbs reflective cycle is a six-phase framework (Figure 22.2) that can be used to learn from an experience. The frameworks phases each have an underpinning question that Sue could ask herself and Sam explains that each of the phases could be used as headings within this final chapter of Sue's dissertation.

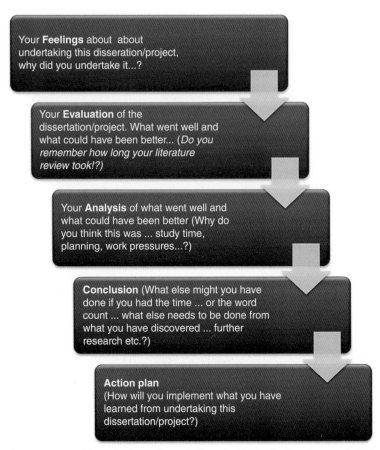

Figure 22.3 Gibbs reflective cycle applied to the final reflective chapter of Sue's dissertation.

Sue looks at Gibbs cycle and says '*I don't get how it fits with my dissertation …* ' So Sam draws out the cycle so that it fits the circumstances of Sue's final chapter (Figure 22.3).

Sue notices that Sam has not included 'description' in his drawing. Sam explains that the description element could be the introduction of this chapter, the way in which Sue begins the chapter and explains to her supervisor what this chapter is about.

'*I think I am getting this …* ', says Sue, '*did you use Gibbs for your Masters thesis?*'

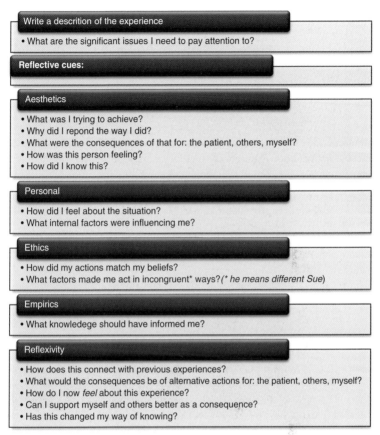

Write a description of the experience

• What are the significant issues I need to pay attention to?

Reflective cues:

Aesthetics

• What was I trying to achieve?
• Why did I repond the way I did?
• What were the consequences of that for: the patient, others, myself?
• How was this person feeling?
• How did I know this?

Personal

• How did I feel about the situation?
• What internal factors were influencing me?

Ethics

• How did my actions match my beliefs?
• What factors made me act in incongruent* ways?(* *he means different Sue*)

Empirics

• What knowledege should have informed me?

Reflexivity

• How does this connect with previous experiences?
• What would the consequences be of alternative actions for: the patient, others, myself?
• How do I now *feel* about this experience?
• Can I support myself and others better as a consequence?
• Has this changed my way of knowing?

Figure 22.4   Johns (1997) model of structured reflection (Johns, 2003).

Johns (1997) model of structured reflection

Sam explains that for his masters he wanted to really explore the process of writing his thesis so he decided to use Johns (1997) model of structured reflection, as illustrated in Johns (2003) (Figure 22.4). Johns model integrates Carper's (1978) *Fundamental ways of knowing* to provide guided cues from which reflection can take place and the practitioner can begin to interpret, critically analyse and understand the situation.

Sam explains that Carper's (1978) *Fundamental ways of knowing* are based upon how, as nurses, we know what we know about ourselves as practitioners; it is the knowledge that informs what we do in our day to day practice.

Aesthetic knowledge is concerned with the 'art' of this situation. Our ability to feel empathy, and in many ways this knowing, is grounded in our subjective reaction to what we see and how we feel about it. So in the case of Sue's dissertation this knowing is how she felt about her project; we know that she was trying to achieve her BSc (Hons)! But what did she really feel? Apprehensive, out of her depth, confused? Or maybe she felt excited, confident or inspired?

Personal knowledge is our attempt to understand ourselves; we need to explore how our cultural and life experiences have shaped us and what judgements we may make about situations or people as a result of these experiences. Personal knowing is about what makes us who we are. For Sue this is what made her decide to undertake this study in the first place; why did she want to be a nurse with a degree and what influenced this decision? What was it about her personal experiences that made her chose to look at the topic she did for her dissertation?

Ethical knowledge is about our morals and the principles we hold and is linked to personal knowing. Ethics of a situation requires us to explore the extent to which we value and respect individuals or ourselves. Sam asks Sue '*why did you want to look at the topic you chose?*' and then a difficult question '*did you suspect that the care that was being given was not as good as it could be?*'

Empirical knowledge relates to evidence, literature and theories that support practice. For Sue this element should be the easiest to describe, as this will relate to the evidence she has established and the knowledge she has gained from undertaking her dissertation.

Reflexivity … '*Well*', says Sam, '*this is the bit where you summarise all of the above. Try not to be too self-conscious but write about … you*'.

Reflexivity is really the point where Sue can really look at 'Sue the person' and, as Bolton (2005) describes, tell the story of how Sue's dissertation journey has changed Sue's sense of self.

Sam says '*tell the story of "Sue the nurse"*'.

'*Thanks Sam.*'

'*OK*', says Sam, '*I just want to add some final cautions here before you begin this chapter*'.

Some final points on reflection

What reflection is NOT:

- A stick with which to beat yourself or others
- A descriptive account
- To be shared if you are uncomfortable/not ready
- To be shared with those who you do not trust
- To be criticised.

Instead Sam tells Sue that reflection should be:
- An opportunity for personal growth and professional development
- Very challenging
- A compassionate, non-judgemental observation of our own experiences.

In conclusion Sam thinks that reflection does transcend other forms of learning and is without a doubt a creator of wisdom.

References

Bolton, G. (2005) *Reflective Practice* (2nd edn). Sage Publications, London.

Carper, B.A. (1978) Fundamental patterns of knowing in nursing. *Advances in Nursing Science*, **1** (1), 13–23.

Dewey, J. (1929) *Experience and Nature*. Grave Press, New York.

Driscoll, J. and Teh, B. (2001) The potential of reflective practice to develop individual orthopaedic nurse practitioners and their practice. *Journal of Orthopaedic Nursing*, **5**, 95–103.

Gibbs, G. (1988) *Learning by Doing: A guide to Teaching and Learning Methods*. Further Education Unit, Oxford Polytechnic, Oxford.

Johns, C. (2003) Opening the Doors of Perception. In: C. Johns and D. Freshwater (eds), *Transforming Nursing through Reflective Practice*. Blackwell Publishing, Oxford.

Johns, C. (2004) Foreword. In S. Tate and M. Stills (eds) *The Development of Critical Reflection in the Health Professions*. Occasional Paper 4, Higher Education Academy, Health Sciences and Practice Subject Centre, London (http://www.health.heacademy.ac.uk/rp/publications/occasionalpaper/occp4.pdf/ (accessed 25 May 2012).

Schon, D. (1983) *The Reflective Practitioner: How Professionals Think in Action*. Basic Books, New York.

Remen, R.N. (1997) *Kitchen Table Wisdom*. Stories That Heal. Riverhead Books, New York.

For further resources for this chapter visit the companion website at

📧 **www.wiley.com/go/glasper/nursingdissertation**

Chapter 23 **Building the architecture of your dissertation**

Alan Glasper[1] and Colin Rees[2]
[1]*University of Southampton, UK*
[2]*University of Cardiff, UK*

Writing your evidence-based practice thesis

1 *Use the decimal notation system*, commonly known as the civil service format, to write each section of your thesis. Although not compulsory, many students writing dissertations find it easier to use the civil service format for delineating the various subsections of their dissertations. Consequently, in **Chapter 1** the main heading of an EBP dissertation might be 1 Writers disease (main heading), followed by 1.1 The incidence of Writers Disease (smaller heading), and then possibly followed by 1.1.1 Gender differences in Writers Disease (small heading) and so on. Still in **Chapter 1**, the next section might be 1.2 The prevalence of Writers Disease, with subsections as above. This might then be followed by 1.3 The management of Writers Disease, in turn followed by 1.4 The role of government policy in managing Writers disease, 1.5 The role of evidence-based practice in the management of Writers Disease, 1.6 Formulating an EBP question pertinent to Writers Disease using the PICO framework. This style of formatting can be used throughout the whole dissertation; hence, Chapter 2 would follow similarly with 2.1, 2.1.1 and so on, 2.2, 2.3 and so on.

Scenario

Sue does not really understand the decimal notation format of report writing and her friend Sam gives her a good suggestion. He asks her to examine any government healthcare report. Sue accesses one of the National Service Frameworks and suddenly it becomes clear to her!

How to Write Your Nursing Dissertation, First Edition. Alan Glasper and Colin Rees.
© 2013 John Wiley & Sons, Ltd. Published 2013 by John Wiley & Sons, Ltd.

2 *Searching the literature and sourcing the evidence.* Many students find this the most technically difficult chapter to write. It is a formulaic chapter and must include a number of subsections to demonstrate that the student has not simply sourced the papers randomly from the Internet. Perhaps because of this, most searching the literature chapters follow the same format. This normally constitutes Chapter 2 of the dissertation and should include:

- Reference to a literature searching method (for example, Timmins and McCabe, 2005).
- Discussion of a hierarchy of evidence in healthcare. What is best and why?
- Navigating the scholarly databases in selecting evidence. What are the bibliographic databases and which have been used? Students should consider using a table. (The sample dissertation hosted on the companion website of this book at www.wiley.com/go/glasper/nursingdissertation provides an example of the chapter architecture required for this element.)
- Searching the literature by hand. Here the student should discuss how hand searching complemented the search of the bibliographic databases.
- Searching the Cochrane (http://ukcc.cochrane.org/) and other eminent data bases (e.g. CRD-centre for reviews and dissemination hosted by The University of York (http://www.york.ac.uk/inst/crd/) and The Joanna Briggs Institute for Evidence Based Nursing (http://www.joannabriggs.edu.au/)).
- Using Grey Literature. It is important to include some reference to the use of grey literature in this element of the dissertation.
- Using expert opinions. Students wishing to gain extra insights into the solving of clinical questions are advised to seek opinions from key informant experts, such as clinical researchers, clinical nurse specialists and consultants. Evidence of correspondence with their key informants can be alluded to in the text with letters and emails being placed in one of the dissertation appendices.
- Using the Internet. It is important to give details of how you have used the Internet search engines, such as Google, Google Scholar and so on, but you must also discuss their strengths and limitations.
- Using health services bench marked practice policy publications, such as government health polices, to source additional evidence is always helpful and a useful inclusion for any dissertation.
- Give details of your database search strategy with key search terms, Boolean logic, wild cards and truncations (students are recommended to consider using a table).

Scenario

Sue and Sam have been getting to grips with searching the literature. One of the lecturers has given them a table of an initial search strategy he used for some work on evaluating clown humour for children in hospital.

Databases searched for the clown humour example
- *AMED 1985–2005*

Search terms: (Laughter/ or clown$ or "Wit and humor"/) AND (child$ or pediatric or paediatric)
- *BNI British Nursing Index 1985–2005*

Search terms: (humour/or clown$ or laughter) AND (child$ or pediatric or paediatric)
- *CINAHL 1982–2005*

Search terms: (Hospitals, Pediatric/ or Child, Hospitalized/) AND (clown$ or laughter)
- *Embase 1980 to 2005 Week 18*

Search terms: (Pediatric hospital/ or Child Hospitalization/) AND (clown$ or laughter)
- *HMIC Health management information consortia 1983–2005*

Search terms: (Humour/ or clown$ or laughter)
- *Medline 1966 to April Week 3 2005*

Search terms: (Laughter therapy/or Laughter/ or "Wit and humor"/ or clown$) AND (Hospitals , pediatric/or Child hospitalized/)
- *Psycinfo 1985 to April Week 4 2005*

Search terms (Humor/ or clown$ or laughter) AND (hospitalized patients or pediatrics)
- *Web of Science 1981–2005*

Search terms: (laughter or clown$) AND (child$ or pediatric or paediatric)
- *ASSIA Applied Social Sciences Index and Abstracts 1987–2005*

Search term: clown$
- *Index of Theses (including Irish section)*

Search terms: clowns or laughter
- *University library catalogue: clowns*
- *British library catalogue: 1) clowns and (therapy or hospital*); 2) laughter and (therapy or hospital*)*

Library of congress: clowns and (therapy or hospital*)
Southampton city library: clowns or laughter
- *Artilcesfirst Database: ArticleFirst Query: kw: therapy and ti: laughter*

- It is important to include a table of the inclusion and exclusion criteria applied.

- Prepare a long short list of papers that have been identified. Students should consider putting this in a table format with author, title, journal and year of publication, the database and a brief outline of the study. The final selection of 3–5 data-driven papers should be double starred** (more for postgraduate and PhD dissertations).
- Accurately list, using the Harvard reference system, your final short list selection of papers.
- Use the 'Savage and Callery grid method' of displaying the primary attributes of the selected papers. (A copy of a Savage and Callery grid is available via the web resource which accompanies this book.)

3 *Critical appraisal.* In this section of the dissertation, which is often Chapter 3, students are advised to include sections pertinent to:
- What is critical appraisal?
- Types of critiquing tools.
- Selection of the critiquing tool(s).
- Following each step of the tool to critique the selected papers. It is recommended that students critique the papers collectively and not one by one.
- It is important to stress that all critiquing tools require readers to investigate the results or data analysis section of the papers they are appraising. For undergraduate dissertations this requires a preliminary understanding and description of the statistics used in the papers. For postgraduate dissertations significantly more detail is required.

4 *The conclusions and implications* of the literature critique are usually formatted as a separate chapter and should include:
- Details pertinent to the value of the research findings for the student's particular field of practice.
- A table showing the strengths and limitations of the studies should be included in this section.
- The students should summarise the evidence from each paper critiqued and weigh up the value of the evidence.

5 *Implementing evidence in practice.* In this section (often the final chapter of the dissertation) students are required to consider how evidence can be introduced into practice. They are asked to write about the barriers or impediments that prevent full implementation of evidence in clinical environments. This includes a number of aspects:
- Managing change in clinical practice; some universities require students to consider change theory.
- The role of leadership in the management of change (students are often required to include the work of the Royal College of Nursing and The Kings Fund, which have been at the forefront of leadership and change

within healthcare settings) (http://www.rcn.org.uk/development/
practice/leadership)
(http://www.kingsfund.org.uk/leadership/)
- Students must consider the barriers to change and, importantly, include fully referenced detail on how to overcome these barriers.

6 *Reflection.* Many universities expect students to use a model of reflection in the final aspect of the dissertation to describe their academic journey.

7 *Using appendices.* Although dissertation markers cannot award marks for appendices, they can judge overall student effort through the quality of appendices. The student can use appendices to ensure that the whole is greater than the sum of the parts. The strict word count applied to dissertations does not apply to appendices and students can use them to place important evidence of their overall effort and furthermore allude to this within the text of individual chapters.

Scenario

Sue and Sam have been contemplating how they can best optimise the appendices facility afforded within the overall dissertation.

Sue has decided to append a full copy of the critiquing tool she has used and Sam is considering appending his correspondences with the range of clinical nurse specialists he has written to during the dissertation journey

---

8 *Using the supervisor.* All students writing a dissertation are advised to use their supervisor wisely, be cognisant of word limits, be fully aware of how the dissertation should be formatted and, importantly, understand the importance of proof reading their work for 'typos and spelling/grammatical errors'.

9 *References.* Students can be penalised up to 10% for reference errors. The crime of reference error is an own goal. Best avoided!

10 *Binding.* Leave at least five working days to allow for binding. (Hot tip: bind a photocopy of the dissertation rather than a copy from a printer as the process of printing often distorts the pages.) NB: dissertations impregnated with tobacco residue may not be marked!

11 *Gaining an academic extension.* Universities are very sympathetic to students who require an extension period to finish their dissertations. This especially applies to students learning beyond registration where job pressure may negatively impact on best laid temporal plans. All universities have procedures to consider student appeals for mitigation or course work extension. However, students are advised to ask for this ahead of time and not on the day the dissertation is scheduled to be submitted!

Scenario

It is summer time and Sue and Sam have just met in the local pub to celebrate their success in being awarded their degrees at the university conferment of awards ceremony. A great result!

Reference

Timmins, F. and McCabe, C. (2005) How to Conduct an effective literature search. *Nursing Standard*, **20** (11), 41–47.

For further resources for this chapter visit the companion website at
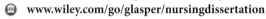   **www.wiley.com/go/glasper/nursingdissertation**

Chapter 24 **Glossary of common research and statistical terms**

Colin Rees[1] and Peter Nicholls[2]
[1]*University of Cardiff, UK*
[2]*University of Southampton, UK*

Scenario

Sue and Sam have found that they share a common difficulty with the language of research. Sue is frequently frustrated that words she feels she is familiar with are given a different interpretation in research. Words like 'significant' and 'random' are not quite the same. She also has a particular problem with the language of statistics. When she reads the methodology and results sections of quantitative articles, she finds the words form a barrier to understanding if the article is of use or not. Sam finds that he in encountering many new words that just leave him baffled. Both are beginning to feel like research is becoming a foreign language to them.

Spending a long time working on your own on your dissertation means that when new and specialised words are encountered there is not always someone available who can quickly explain what they mean. As you read through this book you may have encountered some of these words, and certainly when reading research articles you will identify with the situation described by Sue and Sam.

The aim of this chapter is to provide you with quick access to common terms that form the basic language of research, including essential statistical terms. There are a number of ways you can increase your fluency in these terms:

- Turn to this section each time you encounter a specialised or unfamiliar term and check if it is explained.

How to Write Your Nursing Dissertation, First Edition. Alan Glasper and Colin Rees.
© 2013 John Wiley & Sons, Ltd. Published 2013 by John Wiley & Sons, Ltd.

- In a notebook construct your own 'glossary' of words or terms that seem to be frequently encountered.
- Browse this chapter frequently starting at random and read some of the entries.

Although you may not have thought of reading a chapter like this as any other chapter, it can be useful to browse this chapter while having a break or having a coffee. Read some of the entries that are unfamiliar, or choose words that you feel you know, think how you would define them and then check the entry. In this way your familiarity and understanding of these terms will increase.

It is important in your dissertation to use the right language and to be accurate in the way you explain terms to your readers. This chapter will help you increase your knowledge and understanding of important terminology. Use it often. As usual for a glossary of terms, words are set out in alphabetical order.

A

Accidental sampling: See 'Convenience sampling'.

Action research: Research design that introduces change agreed with those in a setting and then evaluates the outcome, followed by further change and evaluation in a cyclical process. There is no control group. The results are not always transferable because of features of the setting and the people implementing the change.

Aim: This is the statement of what the researcher will try and answer through the collection of data. The aim gives the study direction and purpose. It usually begins with the word 'to' such as 'the aim of this study is to examine the effect of X on Y'.

Anonymity: An important element in research ethics where the identity of a respondent is protected and not revealed. This can encourage people to be more honest and open in replying to questions.

Analysis of Variance (ANOVA): A form of hypothesis testing used to assess the difference in response to two or more treatments or interventions in a wide range of research designs. The non-parametric equivalent to the one-way analysis of variance is the Kruskal–Wallis test. The non-parametric equivalent to a one-way repeated measure analysis of variance is the Friedman test.

Analysis of Covariance (ANCOVA): An extension to the analysis of variance (ANOVA) used to adjust for and assess the effect of one or more variables not controlled in the trial design that may affect outcome, hence analysis of *covariance*.

Audit: Although this often looks like research, this collects data on a measure of performance in a clinical area and compares it to a baseline measure or standard. The information is not transferable to other situations in the same way as research. It also does not increase our understanding of a topic or issue. The main limitation is whether those included in an audit are representative of the total group.

Audit trail: In qualitative research where the researcher provides clear evidence of how the data were broken down from the large amounts of interview or observational data into smaller clusters to provide the main themes for the study. This should be transparent and allow others to follow a similar process leading to similar results.

B

Back chaining: Used in literature searching where the reference section of one article is used to identify other likely articles. Avoid starting this process with an old article as they will take you further into the past to literature that will be less relevant. See also 'Forward chaining'.

Bar graph: A graph style used with categorical or 'nominal' data in which the height of each bar illustrates the relative frequency of each category.

Beneficence: In ethics the obligation of the researcher to ensure that involvement in a study does good rather than harm.

Bias: Relates to an aspect of the design of a study that adversely influences or distorts the results so they are not accurate or representative; for example, asking those attending a sports centre to assess their general fitness level as an indicator of fitness levels in the overall population.

Blinding: See '**Double-blind study**' and '**Masking**'.

Bonferroni correction: When carrying out a large number of statistical tests, applying the Bonferroni correction sets a more demanding level defining statistical significance.

Box plot: A box plot is a graphical representation of data that presents five items of information in the form of a box (**lower quartile**, **median** and **upper quartile**) plus **maximum** and **minimum** values. Some versions identify extreme or outlying values (**outliers**).

C

Causal relationship: A causal relationship or effect goes beyond the effect of one or more treatment variables that may be found to be related to outcome in a randomised controlled trial. To claim causality requires meeting criteria such as strength of association, specificity, timing, intervention response and consistency proposed, among others, by Bradford-Hill.

Cell: Relates to the layout of a table where each square is referred to as a cell.

Chi-squared test (χ^2): Used to assess the statistical significance of the association between categorical variables; for example, males versus females answering 'yes' or 'no' to a question on having undergone cosmetic surgery.

CINHAL: Name of a popular and respected nursing database. The abbreviation stands for Cumulative Index for Nursing and Allied Health Literature.

Closed questions: In interviews or questionnaires a form of asking a question where there is no flexibility in how questions are answered, that is a choice must be made from a list or 'yes/no'. Also called a **'fixed-choice' question**.

Cluster sample: A sampling method where a sampling frame is made up not of individuals but of groupings of individuals, such as those in a named geographical or clinical area. If selected, everyone in that sampling unit is included in the data collection, for example picking so many clinical areas from a list and including all those in the chosen areas in the study.

Coding: In qualitative research a method of analysis where similar words or ideas are grouped under the same heading. This process provides a way of managing large amounts of unstructured information. Also used in quantitative research to allocate a numerical code to ordered categories. Appropriate statistical methods may then be applied to assess association or to compute composite score; for example, 0 for disagree, 1 for neither agree or disagree and 2 for agree.

Concept definition: How a variable or concept is described or defined for the purposes of a study. This increases clarification and allows comparisons with similarly studies. Think of it as a kind of dictionary definition. It is useful to compare different definitions and comment on which you feel is better and why. See also **'operational definition'**.

Confidentiality: In ethics the process of ensuring that privileged information is not accessible to those who should not have access to it.

Confidence interval: A confidence interval is reported when presenting sampled-based estimates of population parameters, most commonly the population mean. In 95% of samples the estimate of the true mean will fall within the reported 95% confidence interval. 99% or other confidence levels may be reported.

Confounding variable: In an experimental study this is a variable not controlled by the researcher that may influence the outcome. It is important to identify these as they may reduce the accuracy of a researcher's claim to have found a relationship between variables.

Contingency table: A visual way of showing the breakdown of one variable by another variable in a table by columns and rows. For example, gender: males and females and wears glasses: 'yes' and 'no'. This is used to identify the level of association or pattern between the variables in the study. Also referred to as a **cross-tabulation**.

Control group: In an experimental study this the group that forms the comparison. It does not have the experimental variable given to the experimental group and is used to see what would have happened without the intervention. It should be identical to the experimental group. Usually, random allocation will achieve this providing the size of the groups is large enough.

Convenience sample (also called an **accidental** or **opportunity sample**): In sampling methods the use of those people who are easily accessible and at the right place at the right time for the purpose of the study. Although they may give a useful indication of results, there may be factors that influence their availability that may have a distorting effect on the results; for example, using patients attending a GP surgery to assess the health level of general population.

Correlation: Correlation is a measure of the association between two interval variables. This is measured by **Pearson's Product Moment Correlation Coefficient**. The non-parametric equivalent is **Spearman's Rank Order Correlation Coefficient**. A correlation does not indicate a 'cause-and-effect' relationship.

Covert observation: Form of observation where data are gathered without the subjects being aware they are part of a study. From an ethical point of view this breaks the rule of informed consent.

Cronbach's alpha: A measure of multiple correlation between the items of a measurement scale reflecting internal consistency or reliability. This gives some confidence in the accuracy of the tool for data collection.

Cross-sectional study: Type of research design that takes the form of a survey where different group are included at one point in time rather than follow the same group over time, for example patients at different points in their treatment.

Critique: Attempt to provide a balanced assessment of a research article that includes an assessment on the quality of the research decisions made during the study. It is important that this is not seen as simply criticising or finding fault with a study.

D

Data: Individual items of information occurring in different forms or **data types** or **levels of measurement**. These include **interval** data, such as physical measurements, **ordinal** data, ordered categories such as levels of symptom severity, and **nominal** data, unordered categories such as used to describe marital status. Individual data items are referred to as **variables**. **Ratio** data arise from the comparison of two interval measures.

Database: Computerised listing of published articles. It is important to use reputable databases to ensure that articles are from peer reviewed journals, that is, that their quality and accuracy has been checked prior to publication. Databases should be listed in your search strategy at the start of a literature review. The same term is also used to describe organised and indexed data held on computer.

Data saturation: In qualitative research when no new themes emerge from the data analysed and further data collection is then stopped.

Demographic data: Personal characteristics of the sample that help to categorise or describe individuals or indicate patterns of interest.

Dependent variable: In randomised controlled trials the variable the researcher is trying to influence, for example level of anxiety or level of pain. It is the outcome measure of an experimental study. The variable that influences it is the independent variable.

Descriptive statistics: Used to summarise data. They may be **measures of central tendency**, such as **mean, mode or median**, or **measures of dispersion**, such as **standard deviation or range**.

Dissertation: An impressive document that marks a happy event in the life of many students. It provides an opportunity to demonstrate your knowledge and skills and make your contribution to nursing knowledge.

Double-blind study: Where neither the subjects in a randomised controlled trial, or those supervising treatment or collecting data, are aware whether an individual is in the experimental or control group. **Triple-blinding** extends this to those responsible for data analysis. This reduces bias in such studies but is not always possible, depending on the nature of the intervention and whether it can be hidden from the individual, for example emersion in water. **Masking** is also used as an alternative term to blinding to mean the same thing.

E

Ethics committee: Body charged with examining research proposals involving 'live subjects' or human tissue and judging if they follow sound ethical principles before permission is given for the study to take place. If an article states that ethical permission was gained, it can be assumed that the major ethical issues or informed consent, assessment of harm, justice and so on have satisfied the ethics committee or it would not have been given permission. The American equivalent is an **Institutional Review Board** or **IRB**.

Ethnographic research: Study design in qualitative research where the researcher spends time in a social setting observing and talking to members of a group with a common 'cultural' identity. The aim is to identify patterns of behaviour and beliefs held by that group. This approach developed from anthropological research. An example would be an ethnographic study of patients in a clinical area for chronic illness that observed what they did and interviewed them about their feelings and beliefs about their condition and its impact on their life.

Experimental research: Type of study that tests relationships between an independent (predictor) and dependent (effect) variable. Individuals are randomly allocated to an experimental or control group. In healthcare, this usually takes the form of a randomised controlled trial (RCT). Some studies do not include one of the key elements in an RCT, such as randomisation, and are termed a '**quasi-experimental**' study.

Equivalence test: The form of hypothesis testing used to demonstrate that treatments are equivalent in their effect. Also known as **non-inferiority** testing. The wording of null and alternative hypotheses are reversed, though the null hypothesis continues to provide the basis for the test.

F

Face validity: An assessment, frequently by experts, that confirms the items in a questionnaire or scale appear relevant to the topic or research question, that is, 'on the face of it' they are appropriate.

Factor analysis: A method of multivariate analysis used to identify underlying dimensions (latent variables), defined by but fewer in number than the variables in the original data set.

Focus group: Type of interview where small groups of people (e.g. 5–8) are brought together by the researcher to discuss their views on a common theme.

Forward chaining: In literature searching using links such as 'cited in' or 'similar studies' in databases to find more recent research of the same type as ones already identified.

Frequency distribution: Common forms include the normal and Poisson distributions. Data distributions may be summarised using histograms or tables that illustrate the relative frequency of each data value.

G

Generalisability: The ability to apply the results of a study to similar settings. The more representative or typical the sample, and the greater control the researcher has used over other possible influences on the outcome, the more generalisable the results.

Grey literature: A source of evidence that has not yet been published. This includes dissertations, theses and conference papers.

Grounded theory: Study design in qualitative research where the researcher provides an explanation or theory that fits the data collected in a study, not just a description. It developed from sociological research methods.

H

Hawthorne effect: Relates mainly to experimental studies where people may act differently in the direction of the desired effect merely because psychologically they feel special to be included in a study and react to their inclusion rather than to anything the researcher is testing. This is similar to *placebo effect* and so forms a threat to validity. This is partly the reason for a control group in such studies.

Heterogeneity: Feature of a sample where there is a diverse range of characteristics. Often used in relation to a non-random sample so they will be reasonably representative of the wider population. This reduces bias. Opposite term is *homogeneity* where the sample is very similar in characteristics.

Hermeneutics: A type of phenomenological qualitative research where an attempt is made to interpret the actions and meanings of those involved in a study. Derived from the role of the Greek god Hermes, who interpreted the messages sent from the gods for those on earth.

Hierarchy of evidence: In evidence-based practice the value put on different sources of evidence depending on the methodology that has created it. The greater the levels of generalisability due to the methodology used, the higher up the hierarchy the source of evidence is placed. A number of hierarchies exist. In many hierarchies the systematic reviews or randomised controlled trials form the top element.

Histogram: A graphical presentation of the frequencies of values of a single continuous variable. Looks similarly to a bar graph but here the bars touch, for example height or blood pressure.

Homogeneity: Feature of a sample where those selected are very similar in relation to key characteristics that may affect outcome.

Hypothesis testing: A probability-based test procedure, most commonly used to assess the probability that an observed outcome (e.g. a difference between means) has occurred by chance. A statistical test is used to compute the probability (**statistical significance**) of the observed difference based on the assumption that the null hypothesis is true. Probabilities less than 0.05 ($p < 0.05$) lead to rejection of the null hypothesis and acceptance of the **alternative hypothesis** that a difference between scores is unlikely to be explained by chance. Probabilities greater than or equal to 0.05 lead to acceptance of the null hypothesis.

I

Inclusion and exclusion criteria: These can be used in two different settings. Firstly, in searching the literature where the kind of literature wanted and not wanted are listed and used to judge whether to include papers. Secondly, as part of sampling where the characteristics of the sample are listed in terms of desirable and undesirable features and then used to select those for the study. In both situations such criteria demonstrate the systematic and logical processes involved and form part of the transparency of high quality work.

Inferential statistics: The process of drawing conclusions about a population based on a sample drawn from that population. It encompasses a wide range of statistical methods, specifically estimation, hypothesis testing and methods of regression analysis.

Independent variable: In randomised controlled trials this is the variable the researcher introduces to test its effect on the dependent variable that forms the outcome measure.

Informed consent: Key ethical principle in research where those taking part in a study must have agreed to do so but only once the details of the study and what will happen to them have been fully explained and understood.

Interviews: Method of data collection in both quantitative and qualitative research designs. Can be face-to-face with individuals or groups, telephone or electronic, for example web based

IRB: Stands for Institutional Review Board and is the American equivalent of a UK Local Research Ethics Committee (**LREC**) ethics committee. Mention of this indicates ethical rigour in an American study.

Instrument: In research methods, it is the method used to measure the outcome of the study, such as questionnaire or pain scale.

J

Judgemental sample: Sampling approach in qualitative studies where the sample is handpicked on the basis of the researcher's judgement of a typical spread of characteristics. Also referred to as a ***purposive sample***.

Justice: Principle of research ethics where there is an obligation to ensure all those included in a study receive the same human rights and respect. This ensures there is no form of discrimination applied to the sample in terms of who has access to which form of intervention.

K

Key informant: In qualitative research those in a study who have a special insight or hold an influential position that is helpful to the aims of the study.

Key word: In literature searching the words used to find likely articles in databases.

L

Level of statistical significance: The level of **probability** applied in **hypothesis testing** which determines the acceptance or rejection of the null hypothesis. Most often set at 0.05 but also reported at the 1% ($p < 0.01$) or 0.1% ($p < 0.001$) levels.

Likert scale: Method of structuring the answers to a question where respondents choose along a scale, for example, from 'strongly agree' to 'strongly disagree' in response to a statement. Each answer is given a numeric value. It is named after the American psychologist Rensis Likert, so 'Likert' always starts with a capital letter.

Literature review: This is an important aspect of the research process, where the study is put within the context of current and past studies, and a prominent part of a dissertation. A key element is the sourcing of good quality research. This should be written as a critical review and not just a summary of what has gone before.

M

Manipulation: Part of the defining criteria of an experimental design where the researcher has the ability to introduce the independent variable and observe the effect on the dependent variable.

Masking: Also called '*blinding*', where an attempt is made in an experimental study to hide or 'mask' whether someone is in the experimental or control group. Both the person receiving an active intervention and the person directly gathering data may differ in their behaviour or estimations if they are aware of an individual's group.

Maximum: The largest value in a data set.

Mean: The arithmetic average calculated by adding together the value of all the units and dividing by the number in the sample.

Measure of location or central tendency: Statistics that describe the middle or other locations in the data set. Examples include the mean, median, mode and percentiles.

Measure of dispersion: Statistics that describe the spread or variability in a data set. Examples include range, maximum, minimum, standard deviation and variance.

Meta-analysis: The consolidation of results from comparable studies identified in the context of a structured literature review (most commonly, a Cochrane Review). The combined results benefit from large sample size and corresponding increase in statistical power to demonstrate the presence or absence of a treatment effect not otherwise evident from individual studies.

Mode: The most common data value.

Median: The middle value of the distribution, in the sense that 50% of data values are less than the median and 50% are greater than the median.

Minimum: The smallest value in a distribution or data set.

Multimodal: The term used to describe a frequency distribution with two peaks or modes. May occur when data from two separate distributions are combined.

N

Naturalistic research: Alternative name for qualitative research and describes a research approach where the researcher does not introduce or manipulate variables as in an experimental design.

Non-maleficence: The ethical principle that researchers should do no harm as a result of their investigations. Usually applies to experimental designs but can apply in all situations where psychological as well as physical harm may be a consequence of the researcher's involvement, including the use of questionnaires.

Non-probability sampling methods: Approaches to sampling such as convenience and purposive sampling, where the extent to which the sample represents the larger population cannot be calculated. This means that generalisations cannot be as readily made as when probability sampling methods have been used

Normal distribution: The symmetrical, bell-shaped frequency distribution that occurs naturally in many physical and other measurements. The associated statistical theory underpins the family of parametric tests. Other common distributions include the Poisson and binomial distributions. The alternative family of non-parametric tests do not require data to follow a known distribution.

Null and alternative hypotheses: Most commonly the null hypothesis takes the form of a statement of no treatment effect or no difference in means. The alternative hypothesis may state that a difference exists or specify the direction of the difference – hence one or two-tailed tests. See **hypothesis testing**.

O

Open questions: In interviews and questionnaires where respondents are not given a list of alternatives to choose from but can answer in their own words. This is the opposite of '*closed questions*'.

Operational definition: In relation to variables this describes how a particular variable is measured in a study, such as using an anxiety scale. It is a way of answering the questions: what 'operationalises' or makes the variable visible.

Opportunity sample: See '**Convenience sample**'.

Outliers: Extreme data values well beyond the expected range. May indicate an error in measurement or data entry, or perhaps the effect of some undiagnosed condition.

P

Paradigm: World view that provides a complete way of looking a topic or situation. In research the two major paradigms are quantitative and qualitative. Each has a different view on the nature of research and the role of the researcher.

Percentiles: These mark each 1% of the distribution, so the median is the fiftieth percentile. Quartiles (25%, 50%, 75%), quintiles (20%, 40%, 60%, 80%), deiles (10%, 20%, 30% etc.) and terciles (33.3%, 66.7%) are also defined.

Phenomenology: Study design in qualitative research where the researcher through in-depth interviews attempts to describe the 'lived experience' of those in a specific situation. The purpose is to develop insights and understanding of how people experience situations. It has developed from phenomenological philosophy and an example would be the lived experience of those with diabetes.

Pilot study: A method of checking the accuracy of the tool of data collection and other methodological aspects of study in a small-scale version or try-out of the study.

Power analysis: The calculation of the sample size that ensures a satisfactory probability of finding a difference statistically significant if it exists. (See **statistical power.**)

Pretest–Posttest design: Type of experimental design, also called 'before and after design', where groups are first measured in relation to the outcome variable. The experimental variable is introduced to one group but not the control group, and the outcome variable for both groups is measured again to see if any difference between the groups can be demonstrated to be due to the experimental variable. Subjects must be randomly assigned or allocated to the two groups for causality to be demonstrated. If the second group is a comparison group where subjects were not randomly allocated by the researcher, causality may not be claimed and the study is described as *quasi-experimental*. The result in this situation can only be correlation.

Probability sampling methods: These produce samples closely mirroring the characteristics of the total population, for example random sampling. These methods are based on the principle of everyone or every unit having an equal chance of being selected.

Prospective study: Study where data exist in the future at the time the study starts. For example, observation of patients over the next two weeks entering the clinical area. This allows greater consistency and accuracy than in the opposite, which is a retrospective study, where the data already exist. The issue is related to the quality control of data. However, sometimes because of ethical issues there can be no other option but to gather data that already exist and a prospective study is not possible.

Population: Those who share a common characteristic and form the total group the researcher wants to explore. Usually, a *sample* is selected to represent this whole group. For example, the population of those on a waiting list for an operation.

Purposive sample: In sampling, a method of handpicking those involved so as to represent a reasonable mix of subjects based on the researcher's knowledge of what is typical in the group. Often used in qualitative research, it is used in more exploratory types of research as it is difficult to generalise from the results. Also called a *judgemental sample*.

Q

Qualitative research: Type of research that focuses on descriptions of situations seen through the eyes of those involved. The findings of such research are in the form of words rather than numbers and these lead to insights into the interpretations and experiences people have of different situations. Common forms under this heading include ethnographic, phenomenological and grounded theory approaches. Generalisations are not possible, although the general themes may occur in other situations. Sometimes referred to as the *interpretative or naturalistic paradigm*.

Quantitative research: Type of research that focuses on the collection of numeric data where the emphasis is on the accuracy of the measurements. The aim of the researcher is to apply the findings to other like situations through generalisation. This is the type of research most favoured in evidence-based practice and includes randomised controlled trials and surveys. Sometimes referred to as the *positivist paradigm*.

Quasi-experimental research: This has the appearance of a randomised controlled trial with an intervention and a control group but the groups have not been randomly allocated, for example where they already exist as groups. This means we cannot rule out other explanations for any differences between the results of the two groups. Instead of a cause-and-effect relationship we can only say there appears to be a correlation. This approach is used when ethically or practically randomisation is difficult.

Questionnaire: Data collection tool that requires respondents to fill in the answers to question either on paper or electronically online. Respondents must have good reading, writing or keyboard skills. As a method, it often suffers from a low proportion of questionnaires returned; this is known as the response rate.

Quota sampling: A non-probability sampling methods in which researchers seek out respondents in relation to a set number per characteristic category, such as age groups or social class groups. This is an attempt to make the results reflect the total population more closely.

R

Randomisation, random allocation: May relate to a sampling method whereby all the members of a study population have an equal chance of being selected for a study. More commonly used to describe the process of *random allocation* of individuals to either an experimental or control group, all individuals meeting the inclusion criteria having an equal chance of being in either group. The aim is to ensure that any other variable that might make a difference to the outcome is equally present in each group. This leaves only the experimental variable the one that could make a difference to the outcome between the groups.

Randomised controlled trial: Experimental research design that compares what happens when an intervention, known as the independent variable (e.g. a form of treatment), is introduced to one group (experimental group) and the results compared with a control group. The control group may have no intervention (sometimes in the form of a placebo) or the 'usual' intervention. The outcome measure is the 'dependent variable' such as level of pain, or level of consciousness. This is a highly valued form of research as it supports the existence of a cause-and-effect relationship between the independent and dependent variables. The method must include random allocation, where each person has an equal chance of being in either the experimental or control group. This reduces the possibility of explaining any differences in the outcome between the groups by some other variable (e.g. differences in pain threshold).

Range: The difference between the maximum and minimum values in a distribution or data set.

Reliability: A key concept applied to the tool of data collection in a study. It refers to the accuracy and consistency of the measurements created by the tool. **Cronbach's alpha** is a measure of the internal consistency of a data collection tool. An indicator of reliability can be the use of a tool used successfully in other studies, or the use of a pilot or try-out of the tool. Inter- and intra-rater reliability are measures of the level of agreement among raters using the tool.

Research design: The type or classification of research study used, such as survey, experimental or qualitative design. It includes a set of decisions and choices, such as the research method, type of data analysis, sampling method and so on appropriate to that design.

Research method: The technique used to collect data in a study. Sometimes referred to as the tool of data collection, examples include questionnaires, interviews and so on.

Response rate: The percentage of those sent a questionnaire that return it, or agreed to take part in a study. Problems occur where the response rate falls below 50%, as those not agreeing or returning a questionnaire outnumber those who do; this may make the results inaccurate as they do not represent the majority. Although is such cases results are rarely dismissed, it is important to remember they do not provide a complete picture of the situation.

Retrospective study: A study collecting data that either already exists somewhere, such as in records, or that relates to a former time or situation, for example last hospital visit. As the data already exist it is difficult to influence them or introduce bias, but it can suffer from a lack of control and so can be of a variable quality. It is the opposite to a ***prospective study***.

Rigour: The care and attention to detail taken by the researcher in designing and carrying out the study so as to produce a high quality study with accurate data and valid conclusions.

S

Sample: Those selected for a study to represent or stand for the wider study population.

Sampling method, sampling plan, or sampling strategy: There are several methods of selecting the sample, some of which are more representative of the population than others. These terms are applied to the methods and the choice made.

Sampling frame: In random sampling the researcher first constructs a numbered list of names or identification numbers of everyone who could be included. This forms the sampling 'frame' in that it encloses all those who could be selected. It is from this list that those entering the study are picked by using computer generated numbers or a table of random numbers to indicate those who correspond with the number selected.

Seminal study: Term used to describe a classic study that started research in a particular topic, or one that has been associated with a breakthrough in the research. In other words, the seed from which others grew. The term is a useful way to refer to an older study to show that you know it is old, but have included it as it has played an important part in the development of the body of knowledge on the topic.

Significant: Term usually applied to a quantitative result that is unlikely to be explained by chance; there is a statistical relationship that suggests a clear relationship. It should not be used as another word for 'important'.

Snowball sample: A method of qualitative sampling where the researcher may start with one or two people and ask them if they can help provide a contact with people in a similar situation. This is then repeated with those contacted in this way. It is used for hard-to-find groups where it is difficult to identify those with the key sample inclusion criteria. Other terms used to describe it are '*chain*' and '*nominated*' and '*network sampling*'; all these terms provide some insight into the method.

Standard deviation (s.d.): A measure of how widely data values are spread around the mean.

Statistical Power: In hypothesis testing, the probability of a finding a true difference statistically significant.

Stratified random sample: Method in random sampling where instead of one large sampling frame, those who could be selected are stratified into groups that will make it easier to selected a meaningful sample mirroring the subdivisions within the larger group.

Structured interviews: In interview studies where everyone is asked the same questions in the same way to achieve standardisation of responses. This makes interview data easier to analyse as questions are often fixed choice where respondents choose option a or b or c and so on.

Survey: Popular method of descriptive research where standardised data are collected from a large group of people. This often involves questionnaires. The problem is to ensure those included are representative of the total group and that the response rate is reasonably high.

T

Tables: Method of displaying numeric data in clearly labelled columns and rows. These should reveal a pattern of the distribution of the results. Look for the pattern that you can see and then read what the researcher identifies as relevant.

Themes: In qualitative research the headings used to group the findings of the study to give them structure and sense. The themes form the main findings of a qualitative study.

t-test: Student's independent t-test is used to test hypotheses concerning the means of two independent groups, for example, the treatment arms in a trial. Student's paired t-test is used to test hypotheses about paired means that arise in before and after research designs or in case-control studies. Both tests require data to be normally distributed. The non-parametric equivalents are the Mann–Whitney U test and the Wilcoxon Signed Rank test respectively. All of these are important ways of processing numerical date to allow conclusions to be drawn from them.

Triangulation: Usually refers to an attempt to reduce the disadvantages of any one method of data collection by using more than one method, for example observation and interviews. This may increase the validity of the findings but will increase the time and costs involved.

Type 1 and Type 2 errors: Since hypothesis testing is probability based, a **Type I error** occurs when the researcher wrongly concludes that a difference exists when there is none and a **Type 2 error** occurs when a researcher concludes that there is no difference when one does exist.

U

Unstructured interviews: In qualitative research interviewing where broad questions are used in a flexible and non-standardised way. The aim is to ensure that information and its relevance are determined by the participant and they are encouraged to follow what they see as important in a free flowing way. The interviewer may add prompts such as 'tell me more about that' or 'how do you mean?'

Unstructured observations: In qualitative research a method of trying to avoid looking for predetermined activities or events and instead being open to whatever shows itself during the course of observation.

V

Validity: The accuracy of the results in terms of whether the data describe or are an accurate representation of what the researcher wanted to measure. For example, has pain level been measured or is it really the level of anxiety?

Variable: the elements in a study that form the interest of the researcher. In experimental studies there will be both a dependent variable, which is the outcome measure, and the independent variable, which is what the researcher introduces and controls to bring about a desired effect on the dependent variable.

Variance: A measure of squared differences about the mean.

Section 8

Don't forget to go to www.wiley.com/go/glasper/nursingdissertation for:

- Seven additional chapters
- Summaries of each chapter in the book
- A range of tools and frameworks
- Sample documents to assist you writing your dissertation
- Useful reference links
- Reference lists for each chapter.

Index

abstracts
    critical appraisal 143, 149, 178–9
    learning outcomes 19–20
    publishing dissertations 229–30,
      231–4
    quantitative research 121–3
    of reviews of effects 68
    time management 97, 99
academic extensions 254
ACCN *see* Association of Chief
    Children's Nurses
acknowledgements sections 20,
    97, 99
action research 44
active reading 105–6, 141–3
aesthetic knowledge 203, 247–8
Allied and Complementary Medicine
    Database (AMED) 61, 252
allocation concealment 171–3
AMED *see* Allied and Complementary
    Medicine Database
analysis understanding 142
anonymity 190
appendices 18, 21, 254
applicability 197
application to practice 131
Applied Social Sciences Index and
    Abstracts (ASSIA) 61, 252
assessment guidelines 14–15
ASSIA *see* Applied Social Sciences Index
    and Abstracts

Association of Chief Children's Nurses
    (ACCN) 75, 188–91
auditability 154
authorship 18

background sections
    critical appraisal 143, 148, 151, 153,
      178, 178–80, 188–9
    learning outcomes 19
BARRIERS scale 43–4
before and after studies 45
Belgian Health Care Knowledge Centre
    (KCE) 91
best evidence 40–51
    approaches 56
    barriers to use of research
      evidence 42–4
    bibliographic databases 59–62
    Cochrane Library 66–9
    dissertation architecture 251
    encouraging use of research
      evidence 45–9
    evidence base for practice 40–42
    exploring and refining
      questions 55–8
    grey literature 64
    identifying search words 58
    implementation strategies 200–202
    journal literature 65–6
    library service support 70–71
    models and frameworks 46–9

How to Write Your Nursing Dissertation, First Edition. Alan Glasper and Colin Rees.
© 2013 John Wiley & Sons, Ltd. Published 2013 by John Wiley & Sons, Ltd.

best evidence (*cont'd*)
  RCN information literacy
    competencies 72–5
  research-based information 40–42
  search strategies 62–5
  searching for research articles 59–62
  sourcing 55–76
  topic selection 56
  web resources 69–70
best practice 198–201
bias 181
bibliographic databases 59–62, 251–3
bibliographies 80
binding dissertations 97, 254
blinding 171–3
block randomisation 169–70
BNI *see* British Nursing Index
Boolean logic 63
British Journal of Neuroscience Nursing 238
British Journal of Nursing 236, 238–9
British Journal of Occupational Therapy 238
British Medical Journal 147
British Nursing Index (BNI) 59, 61–3, 252
Bullock and Batten's Planned Change Model 210, 212

can I prove it? approach 56
Care Quality Commission (CQC) 36, 218–19
CASP *see* Critical Appraisal Skills Programme
categorical variables 183
cause-and-effect relationships 119–20
Centre for Evidence Based Medicine (CEBM) 33–4
change management theory 197, 206–7, 209–12, 253–4
charitable trusts 71, 78
CINAHL *see* Cumulative Index to Nursing and Allied Health Literature
civil service format 250
CLAHRC *see* Collaborations for Leadership in Applied Health Research and Care

clinical effectiveness
  background and history 23–8
  contribution of nursing profession 25–6
  definitions and characteristics 29–32
  dissertation guidelines 38
  improving healthcare 34–8
  PDSA cycle and LEAN thinking 36–7
  sourcing evidence 26–7
  see also evidence-based practice
clinical mindlines 42
clinical trials 68
Cochrane Hierarchy of Evidence 170
Cochrane Library 66–9
Cochrane Reviews 67
coding systems 106
Collaborations for Leadership in Applied Health Research and Care (CLAHRC) 45–6
comprehensive understanding 142
computer referencing packages 84
conclusions sections
  critical appraisal 145, 150–152, 155, 179, 185, 191
  dissertation architecture 253
  learning outcomes 19–21
  publishing dissertations 241
  quantitative research 123
conferences 229–35
confidence intervals 175–6
confidentiality 75
consent *see* informed consent
consistency of style 97, 99
CONSORT Statement (2010) 172
contents pages 20, 99
controlled trials 68
Cooksey Report 46
correlational surveys 117–18
CQC *see* Care Quality Commission
creating interest 233–4
credibility 197
critical analysis
  learning outcomes 15–16, 21
  reading skills 142
  study skills 102–3, 104–5
critical appraisal 7–10
  applying a critiquing tool 145–7

commencing a critique 140
Crombie model 139–40, 147
definitions and characteristics 138–9
dissertation architecture 253
evidence-based practice 26, 33–4
initial read and review of journal
        paper 141–3
interrogating research papers 137–57
learning outcomes 15–16, 18–19
marking criteria 12
Parahoo model 139–40, 149–51,
        177–86
points to consider about a
        paper 143–5
preparing long/short lists 140–141
qualitative research 148–9, 152–5,
        158–65
quantitative research 139, 148, 151–2,
        166–76
randomised controlled trials 139,
        148, 166–76
Rees model 139–40, 151–5, 187–93
Savage and Callery grids 146–7
selecting appraisal tools 139–40
strengths and limitations 156, 184–5,
        187–8
study design 179–82, 189
see also Critical Appraisal Skills
        Programme
Critical Appraisal Skills Programme
        (CASP)
allocation of participants 171
best evidence 74
blinding 171–3
critiquing frameworks 147–9
data analysis 163
focused and answerable
        questions 167–8
follow-up and data collection 173
important outcomes and application
        of results 176
intention to treat analysis 173
presentation of data 174–5
qualitative research 148–9, 158–65
quantitative research 168–70
randomised controlled trials 139,
        148, 166–76

reflection 164–5
research findings 163–4
screening questions 159–60
selecting appraisal tools 139–40
supervision 110, 112
value of the research 164
critical reading 10, 141–3
Crombie model 139–40, 147
Cumulative Index to Nursing and Allied
        Health Literature (CINAHL) 59,
        61–4, 252
curriculum vitae (CV) 230, 241

data analysis
critical appraisal 150, 163, 182–3
learning outcomes 21
qualitative research 130, 132
data collection
critical appraisal 151, 153–4, 162,
        173, 181–2, 189–90
evidence-based practice 26
implementation strategies 220
learning outcomes 15, 19
qualitative research 127–31
quantitative research 115–16
data extraction grids 104–6
data presentation
clinical effectiveness 26
critical appraisal 152, 154, 174–5,
        183–5, 191
qualitative research 130
databases 59–62, 103–4, 251–3
date restrictions 64
deadlines *see* submission deadlines
decimal notation system 250
decision making 201–4
decision trails 154
Delphi instruments 189–91
Deming cycle 36–7
demographic data 183
Department of Health (DH)
best evidence 42, 45–6
clinical effectiveness 29
critical appraisal 188
grey literature 78
implementation strategies 214–16
dependent variables 118–19

descriptive surveys 117–18
developing practice *see* implementation strategies
Dewey, John 243
DH *see* Department of Health
difference trials 176
discussion with peers 107
discussion sections
  critical appraisal 145, 150, 164–5, 184–5
  learning outcomes 21
  publishing dissertations 240–241
  quantitative research 123
dissemination strategies
  clinical effectiveness 27, 32
  implementation strategies 197, 199–202
  learning outcomes 19–21
dissertation architecture 250–255
dissertation features 8–9
dissertation timetables 99
documentary methods 129
double blind trials 172
drafts 10
driver diagrams 221–2

e-journals 66
EBP *see* evidence-based practice
Economic Evaluation Database 68–9
Edinburgh post-natal depression scale 32
education 43, 45
Eight-Step Model 212–14
electronic learning platforms 10
EMBASE 61, 68, 252
empirical knowledge 203, 247–8
Enhanced Diplomas 1
equivalence limits 175
ethical knowledge 203
ethics 7
  best evidence 74–5
  blinding 171–2
  critical appraisal 144, 152, 154, 162–3, 171–2, 182, 190
  implementation strategies 204
  qualitative research 130

quantitative research 130
reflection 247–8
ethnography 128–9, 153
evidence-based practice (EBP)
  background and history 23–8
  best evidence 40–51, 72–5
  contribution of nursing profession 25–6
  definitions and characteristics 33–4
  dissertation architecture 250–255
  dissertation guidelines 14–22
  qualitative research 132
  quantitative research 115
  research questions 86–92
  rigour of evidence 34–5
  sourcing evidence 26–7
experimental research 117
expert opinions 251
extensions 254
eye-ball switch approach 56

feedback
  planning a dissertation 10
  referencing 80
  supervision 110
field diaries 129
field searches 63
file management 106–7
Fisher exact test 183
fittingness 154
focus of studies 143, 151–3, 188
follow-up questions 128, 173
Force Field Analysis 206–7
formative proposals 16
formatting a dissertation 97, 99
formulating questions 26
Framing the Nursing and Midwifery Contribution (DH, 2008) 216
free text searches 62
Fundamental ways of knowing (Carper) 247

Gantt charts 9, 97, 109–10
generalisability 131–2, 185
generalist articles 238–9
Gibbs reflective cycle 245–6

Google/Google Scholar 62, 79, 251
governance 7
graduate attributes 7
grey literature 64, 77–9, 251
grids 104–6, 146–7
grounded theory 153
group inertia 207
guidelines
 assessment 14–15
 clinical effectiveness 31–2
 dissertation contents and
  presentation 17–18
 module assignment 11–12

Harvard system 80, 82–4
HASS *see* Home Accident Surveillance
 System
Health Foundation 38
Health Information Resources 60–61, 70
Health Technology Assessment
 Database 68–9
Healthcare Management Information
 Consortium (HMIC) 61, 64,
 78, 252
HEFC *see* Higher Education Funding
 Council
here we go again approach 56
*High Impact Actions for Nursing and
 Midwifery; The Essential Collection*
 (DH, 2010) 216, 219–22
High Quality Care for All (DH, 2008)
 216
Higher Education Funding Council
 (HEFC) 42
highlighter pens 142, 145–6, 166
HMIC *see* Healthcare Management
 Information Consortium
Home Accident Surveillance System
 (HASS) 88
hypotheses 143, 150, 180
hypothesis testing 56

impediments to change 205–6
implementation strategies 197–226
 best evidence 40–51
 best practice 198–201

change management theory 197,
 206–7, 209–12, 253–4
critical appraisal 152, 155, 164,
 176, 192
dissemination of research 197,
 199–202
dissertation architecture 253–4
Eight-Step Model 212–14
evidence-based medicine 34
Force Field Analysis 206–7
Government policy guidance 216–22
impediments to change 205–6
knowledge and experience 203
leadership 197, 202, 214–16, 219,
 253–4
learning outcomes 19–21
level of evidence 200–201
Lewin's Force Field Analysis 206–7
organisational culture 199–202,
 208–9
Planned Change Model 210, 212
potential barriers to implementation
 of change 199–202, 205–9
publishing dissertations 241
quality 218–19
review and evaluation of effectiveness
 of change 212–14
SMART objectives 210, 213, 221
social movement model 222–3
stakeholder resistance 206–8
Three-Step Model 209–11
using and applying evidence in
 practice 198–205
independent variables 118–19
inductive approaches 129
informal communication 41
information literacy competencies 72–5
information management 75
information retrieval 7
informed consent 162–3
Institute for Health Improvement 38
Institute for Innovation and
 Improvement 38
integrating evidence 26–7
intention to treat analysis (ITT) 173
inter-library requests 66

International Centre for Allied Health
  Evidence 139
international conferences 232
International Standard Book Numbers
  (ISBN) 77
interprofessional relationships 43, 45–6
interviews 128–9, 132
introduction chapters 19–20
ISBN *see* International Standard Book
  Numbers
ITT *see* intention to treat analysis

Joanna Briggs Institute (JBI)
  framework 31, 48–9
Johns, Christopher 242–3, 247–8
Johns model of structured
  reflection 247–8
Journal of Advanced Nursing 236, 238
Journal of Clinical Nursing 236
Journal of Health Care Management 238
journal literature 65–6
journal publishing 229–30, 235–41

KCE *see* Belgian Health Care Knowledge
  Centre
keyword searches 62
King's Fund 71, 78, 253–4
knowing-in-action 243
knowing yourself 103–6
knowledge transfer *see* dissemination
  strategies
Knowledge-to-Action (KTA)
  framework 48–9
Kotter's Eight-Step Model 212–14
Kruskal Wallis test 183
KTA *see* Knowledge-to-Action

language restrictions 64
leadership
  clinical effectiveness 36
  implementation strategies 197, 202,
    214–16, 219, 253–4
  learning outcomes 15
LEAN thinking 36–7
learning outcomes 11–12, 15–16,
  18–22
level of evidence 200–201

Lewin's Force Field Analysis 206–7
Lewin's Three-Step Model 209–11
library service support 70–71, 252
limitations of study sections 180
linear figures 58
literacy competencies 72–5
literature reviews
  best evidence 60
  critical appraisal 149, 179–80
  dissertation architecture 251
  learning outcomes 15, 20
  publishing dissertations 240
  research questions 90–92
  study skills 103–4
  time management 97–8
lived experience 126, 128
local conferences 232
local implementation 197
long short lists 140–141

managing information 75
Mann-Whitney U-test 183
marking criteria 11–12
Mayo Clinic 32
measurement 27, 32
medical early warning system
  (MEWS) 32
MEDLINE 61–4, 68–9, 252
Methodology Register 68–9
methodology sections
  critical appraisal 143–4, 162–3,
    191–2
  quantitative research 121–2
MEWS *see* medical early warning
  system
mind maps 58
minimal important clinical
  difference 174
misunderstandings 206
modified Yale Preoperative Anxiety
  Scale (mYPAS) 181–2
module assignment guidelines
  11–12
motivation to publish 230–231
movement stage 209–11
mYPAS *see* modified Yale Preoperative
  Anxiety Scale

national conferences 232
National Health Service (NHS)
  best evidence 45–6, 60–61, 68–71
  clinical effectiveness 30
  critical appraisal 139, 176, 189–92
  implementation strategies 198–200,
    214, 216–17, 219–22
National Institute for Health and
  Clinical Excellence (NICE) 31, 36,
  218
National Institute for Health Research
  (NIHR) 45–6
NHS *see* National Health Service
NHS Direct 176
NHS Quality Improvement Scotland
  (NHS QIS) 30
NICE *see* National Institute for Health
  and Clinical Excellence
Nightingale, Florence 25–6
NIHR *see* National Institute for Health
  Research
NMC *see* Nursing and Midwifery
  Council
non-blinding 172
Nurse Education Today 238
Nursing and Midwifery Council
  (NMC) 7, 23–4, 36, 73, 217
nursing process model 244
Nursing Roadmap for Quality, The (DH,
  2010) 215–19
Nursing Standard 238
Nursing Times 238–9

objectives 143, 150, 180
observation bias 181
observational studies 129, 132, 180–182
OMRU *see* Ottawa Model of Research
  Use
organisational culture 15, 199–202,
  208–9
organisational support 43, 45–6
Ottawa Model of Research Use
  (OMRU) 47

Parahoo model 177–86
  conclusions and
    recommendations 179, 185

critiquing framework 149–51, 178–9
  data analysis 182–3
  discussion sections 184–5
  literature reviews/
    background 178–80
  research funding 186
  research questions 180
  results sections 179, 183–4
  selecting appraisal tools 139–40
  study design 179–82
PARiHS *see* Promoting Action on
  Research Implementation in Health
  Services
parochial self-interest 206
patient data 75
PDSA *see* Plan-Do-Study-Act
peer review 62, 103–4, 140
personal development 6
personal knowledge 203, 247–8
phenomenology 128, 153
phrase searches 63
Picker Institute Europe 30
PICO model 26, 86–90, 140, 250
pilot studies 189
placebos 118
plagiarism 75
Plan-Do-Study-Act (PDSA) cycle 36–7,
  210–211, 221–2
Planned Change Model 210, 212
population, intervention, comparison,
  outcome *see* PICO model
PowerPoint presentations 234–5
preliminary understanding 142
presentation of data
  clinical effectiveness 26
  critical appraisal 152, 154, 174–5,
    183–5, 191
  qualitative research 130
presentation papers 229–30, 234–5
printed journals 66
prioritisation 106
problem solving 7, 107, 202
professional development 6
project management 7
Promoting Action on Research
  Implementation in Health Services
  (PARiHS) 47–8

proofreading 18
proposals 16
prospective observational
    studies 180–182
PsycINFO 61, 64, 252
publishing dissertations 229–41
    abstracts 229–30, 231–4
    adapting a dissertation for
        publication 239–41
    choosing the right conference 231–2
    conferences 229–35
    formulating a title and creating
        interest 233–4, 236–8
    journal papers 229–30, 235–41
    motivation 230–231
    planning and preparation 235–6
    presentation papers 229–30, 234–5
    reviewing journal guidelines 236
    selecting what to present 232–3
    style of presentation 234–5
    submission procedures 234
    targeting the right journal 238–9

QAA see Quality Assurance Agency
QOF see Quality Outcomes Framework
qualitative research 126–33
    comparison with quantitative
        research 115–17, 129–31
    critical appraisal 148–9, 152–5, 158–65
    definitions 127
    ethnography 128–9, 153
    grounded theory 129, 153
    key elements 129–31
    limitations 132
    lived experience 126, 128
    phenomenology 128, 153
    strengths 131–2
    study design 128–9, 153
quality 218–19
Quality Assurance Agency (QAA) 4, 6
Quality Outcomes Framework
    (QOF) 36
quantitative research 115–25
    comparison with qualitative
        research 115–17, 129–31
    critical appraisal 151–2, 166–76

definitions 116–17
    establishing quantitative nature of
        study 115–17
    experimental approaches 117
    key elements 120–123, 129–31
    limitations 124
    quasi-experimental approaches 117
    reasons for choosing 117
    strengths 120, 124
    study design 117–20, 151,
        168–70, 174
    surveys 117–18
    see also randomised controlled trials
quasi-experimental research 117
questionnaires 128
questions see research questions

randomisation techniques 118–19,
    169–70, 172–3
randomised controlled trials (RCT)
    best evidence 45
    critical appraisal 139, 148, 166–76,
        181, 185
    quantitative research 116, 117, 120
    supervision 110
Rapid Critical Appraisal 26
RCN see Royal College of Nursing
RCT see randomised controlled trials
readability 152, 155, 191–2
reading skills 103–6, 141–3
recommendations 150–152,
    185, 191
Rees model 187–93
    background, focus and aims
        188–9
    critiquing framework 151–5,
        187–8
    data collection, sampling and
        presentation 189–91
    implications for practice 192
    readability 191–2
    results, conclusions and
        recommendations 191
    selecting appraisal tools 139–40
    strengths and limitations 187–8
    study design 189

referencing 80–85
  computer referencing
    packages 84
  dissertation architecture 254
  guidelines 18, 21
  Harvard system 80, 82–4
  study skills 106
  Vancouver system 80–82
reflection 242–9
  critical appraisal 141–3, 164–5
  dissertation architecture 254
  frameworks and models 244–8
  Gibbs reflective cycle 245–6
  Johns model of structured
    reflection 247–8
  learning outcomes 15
  nursing process model 244
  theories and processes 242–4
  what reflection is and isn't 248–9
reflexivity 162, 164, 247–8
refreezing stage 209–11
reliability 119
report writing 7
research-based information 40–42
research contracts 109
research funding 42, 151, 186
research methods 4–6, 26
  see also methodology sections
research questions 86–92
  best evidence 55–8
  critical appraisal 150, 180
  exploring and refining 55–8
  focused and answerable questions 89,
    167–8
  formulating 26
  identifying search words 58
  PICO model 26, 86–90
  SPICE model 86, 90–92
restricted searches 64
results sections
  critical appraisal 144–5, 150, 152,
    155, 163–4, 174–5, 179,
    183–4, 191
  quantitative research 122–3
returning to education 101
returns on investments (ROI) 222

revisions 10, 18, 97–8
Road Map approach 56
ROI see returns on investments
Royal College of Medicine (RCM) 36
Royal College of Nursing (RCN) 4–5,
  29–30, 36, 48, 71–5, 218

sampling methods
  critical appraisal 152, 154, 160–162,
    174, 182, 190
  qualitative research 129–31
Savage and Callery grids 146–7
Schon, D. 243
SCOPUS database 59
Scottish Intercollegiate Guidelines
  Network (SIGN) 31, 36, 139
screening questions 159–60
scurvy 25
search engines 103–4
search strategies 62–5
search words 58
self-interest 206
self-knowledge 103–6
self-reflection see reflection
self-report data 132
service users 30
setting, perspective, intervention,
  comparison, evaluation see SPICE
  model
settings for studies 182
SF-36 health measure 32
sharing knowledge see dissemination of
  research
short lists 140–141
SIGN see Scottish Intercollegiate
  Guidelines Network
significance tests 119
single blind trials 172
skim reading 142
SMART objectives 210, 213, 221
social movement model 222
specialist articles 238–9
speed reading 142
spell-checking 10, 18
SPICE model 86, 90–92, 140
stakeholder resistance 206–8

statistical tools
    critical appraisal 145, 174–6, 183
    qualitative research 130
    quantitative research 119
structured reflection 247–8
study aims 143, 150–151, 153,
        178–80, 189
study design
    critical appraisal 150–151, 153,
        160–162, 179–82, 189
    implementation strategies 200–201
    qualitative research 128–9, 153
    quantitative research 117–20, 151,
        168–70, 174
study questions *see* research questions
study skills 101–7
    critical analysis 102–3, 104–5
    data extraction grids 104–6
    discussions with peers and problem
        solving 107
    file management 106–7
    key skills for dissertations 102–3
    knowing yourself 103–6
    organisation 106–7
    prioritisation 106
    reading skills 103–6
    returning to education 101
subject searches 62
subject thesauruses 62–3
submission deadlines 11, 17, 96, 97, 99
submission procedures 234
summative proposals 16
supervision 8, 16–17, 108–12
    additional support 111
    agreeing a working pattern 109
    anticipating and preventing
        problems 109
    dissertation architecture 254
    distance supervision 110–111
    getting started 108
    resources 112
    study skills 107
    time management 109–10
surveys 117–18
Swiss Cheese approach 56

systematic reviews
    best evidence 67
    critical appraisal 170
    implementation strategies 200–201
    quantitative research 120

Three-Step Model 209–11
time management 9–11, 95–100
    dissertation as an opportunity
        95–6
    dissertation timetables 99
    frame of mind 96–8
    making space for a dissertation 96
    managing other activities 96–7, 98
    supervision 109–10
titles
    critical appraisal 149, 178
    learning outcomes 20
    publishing dissertations 233–4
to-do lists 106
tolerance to change 206
topic selection 16, 56
transferability 155
transferable skills 7
transformational leadership 214–15
trigger points 235
TRIP database 31
triple blind trials 172
truncation searches 63
type II errors 184

unfreezing stage 209–11

Vancouver system 80–82
VAS *see* visual analogue scale
viewpoint 130
vision of the future 213
visual analogue scale (VAS) 181, 183

web resources 69–70, 78–9, 251
Web of Science 252
wildcard searches 63

Yale Preoperative Anxiety Scale
    (YPAS) 181–2